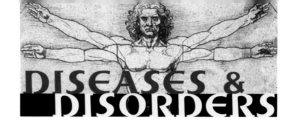

Tuberculosis

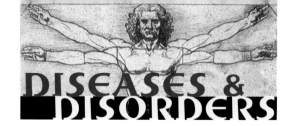

Tuberculosis

Titles in the Diseases and Disorders series include:

Acne
AIDS
Alzheimer's Disease
Anorexia and Bulimia
Anthrax
Arthritis
Asthma
Attention Deficit Disorder
Autism
Bipolar Disorder
·Birth Defects
Brain Tumors
Breast Cancer
Cerebral Palsy
Chronic Fatigue
  Syndrome
Cystic Fibrosis
Deafness
Diabetes
Down Syndrome
Dyslexia
The Ebola Virus
Epilepsy
Fetal Alcohol Syndrome
Flu
Food Poisoning

Headaches
Heart Disease
Hemophilia
Hepatitis
Leukemia
Lou Gehrig's Disease
Lyme Disease
Mad Cow Disease
Malaria
Measles and Rubella
Meningitis
Multiple Sclerosis
Obesity
Ovarian Cancer
Parkinson's Disease
Phobias
SARS
Schizophrenia
Sexually Transmitted
  Diseases
Sleep Disorders
Smallpox
Strokes
Teen Depression
Toxic Shock Syndrome
West Nile Virus

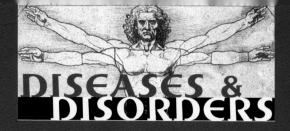

DISEASES & DISORDERS

Tuberculosis

Toney Allman

LUCENT BOOKS

An imprint of Thomson Gale, a part of The Thomson Corporation

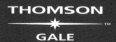

Detroit • New York • San Francisco • New Haven, Conn. • Waterville, Maine • London

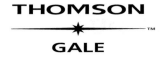

© 2007 Thomson Gale, a part of The Thomson Corporation.

Thomson and Star Logo are trademarks and Gale and Lucent Books are registered trademarks used herein under license.

For more information, contact:
Lucent Books
27500 Drake Rd.
Farmington Hills, MI 48331-3535
Or you can visit our Internet site at http://www.gale.com

LIBRARY OF CONGRESS CATALOGING-IN-PUBLICATION DATA

Allman, Toney.
  Tuberculosis / by Toney Allman.
    p. cm. — (Diseases and disorders series)
  Includes bibliographical references and index.
    Contents: What is tuberculosis?—Deadly mystery—The disease that fought back—Combating TB in the First World—TB warriors for the Third World.
      ISBN-13: 978-1-59018-968-9 (hard cover : alk. paper)
      ISBN-10: 1-59018-968-X (hard cover : alk. paper)
  1. Tuberculosis—Juvenile literature. I. Title. II. Series: Diseases and disorders series.
RA644.T7A397 2006
614.5'42—dc22

                                                                 2006011703

Printed in the United States of America

Table of Contents

"The Most Difficult Puzzles Ever Devised"

Charles Best, one of the pioneers in the search for a cure for diabetes, once explained what it is about medical research that intrigued him so. "It's not just the gratification of knowing one is helping people," he confided, "although that probably is a more heroic and selfless motivation. Those feelings may enter in, but truly, what I find best is the feeling of going toe to toe with nature, of trying to solve the most difficult puzzles ever devised. The answers are there somewhere, those keys that will solve the puzzle and make the patient well. But how will those keys be found?"

Since the dawn of civilization, nothing has so puzzled people—and often frightened them, as well—as the onset of illness in a body or mind that had seemed healthy before. A seizure, the inability of a heart to pump, the sudden deterioration of muscle tone in a small child—being unable to reverse such conditions or even to understand why they occur was unspeakably frustrating to healers. Even before there were names for such conditions, even before they were understood at all, each was a reminder of how complex the human body was, and how vulnerable.

While our grappling with understanding diseases has been frustrating at times, it has also provided some of humankind's most heroic accomplishments. Alexander Fleming's accidental discovery in 1928 of a mold that could be turned into penicillin has resulted in the saving of untold millions of lives. The isolation of the enzyme insulin has reversed what was once a death sentence for anyone with diabetes. There have been great strides in combating conditions for which there is not yet a cure, too. Medicines can help AIDS patients live longer, diagnostic tools such as mammography and ultrasounds can help doctors find tumors while they are treatable, and laser surgery techniques have made the most intricate, minute operations routine.

This "toe-to-toe" competition with diseases and disorders is even more remarkable when seen in a historical continuum. An astonishing amount of progress has been made in a very short time. Just two hundred years ago, the existence of germs as a cause of some diseases was unknown. In fact, it was less than 150 years ago that a British surgeon named Joseph Lister had difficulty persuading his fellow doctors that washing their hands before delivering a baby might increase the chances of a healthy delivery (especially if they had just attended to a diseased patient)!

Each book in Lucent's Diseases and Disorders series explores a disease or disorder and the knowledge that has been accumulated (or discarded) by doctors through the years. Each book also examines the tools used for pinpointing a diagnosis, as well as the various means that are used to treat or cure a disease. Finally, new ideas are presented—techniques or medicines that may be on the horizon.

Frustration and disappointment are still part of medicine, for not every disease or condition can be cured or prevented. But the limitations of knowledge are being pushed outward constantly; the "most difficult puzzles ever devised" are finding challengers every day.

A Renewed Battle Against an Old Enemy

Two billion people—one third of the world's population—are infected with tuberculosis, and 2 million die of the disease every year. This is true even though TB is now a curable disease. Tuberculosis can endanger anyone, in any country, but TB epidemics are the gravest threat to those who cannot obtain the correct medicines or commit to prolonged treatment. This problem is most serious in poor Third World countries; 90 percent of infections and deaths from tuberculosis occur in these nations.

Tuberculosis still exists in developed countries such as the United States but it is not nearly as common as in the developing nations of the Third World. In these nations, TB infections rage in even greater proportions today than they have in the past. Several factors are responsible for this increase, including poverty, the lack of modern treatment methods, and the AIDS epidemic. Diseases of all kinds are usually more prevalent in poor communities. Malnutrition is a common problem among impoverished people, and a malnourished body cannot fight off infection the way a healthy body would. This is one reason why disesases such as TB can gain a foothold in poor communities. Then, once present, such diseases spread more easily because poor people usually have limited or no access to medical care. AIDS, which breaks down the body's natural

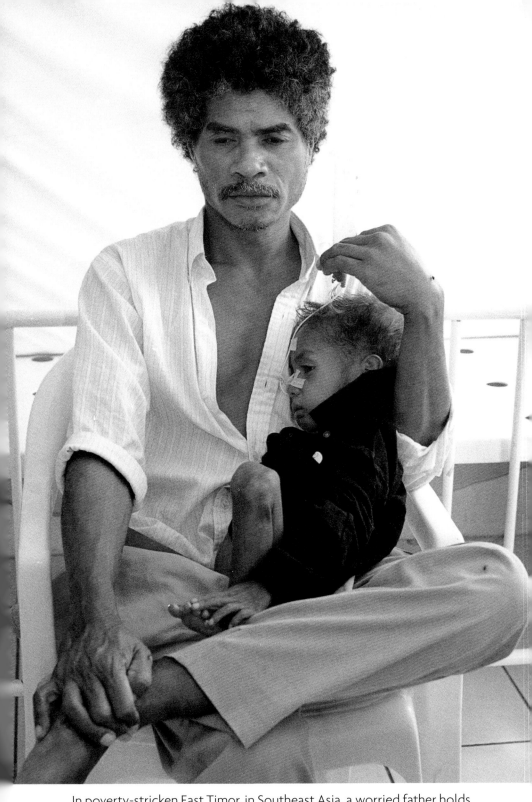

In poverty-stricken East Timor, in Southeast Asia, a worried father holds his three-year-old son, who is afflicted with tuberculosis.

defenses against infection, is now a huge problem in some of the world's poorest nations. The AIDS epidemic has created even more fertile ground for the spread of tuberculosis.

Tuberculosis is a difficult disease to cure because treatment under such conditions is complicated and typically requires many months. Most TB experts believe that what the world needs most is a new, inexpensive drug that can cure or prevent tuberculosis. Although research is ongoing, no new TB drugs have been developed in decades. This situation not only leads to terrible suffering in some parts of the world, it also poses a threat of even more vicious and widespread epidemics in the future.

Scientists have identified new strains of TB that can resist many of the drugs used most often for treatment. Experts predict that if TB is not contained and controlled, it is only a matter of time before a strain of TB that can resist every available tuberculosis medicine develops. This in turn could lead to epidemics of unimaginable strength in every part of the world. As tuberculosis expert Lee B. Reichman says, TB is a timebomb that threatens "all of us who live in the world and breathe its

Government tuberculosis researchers appear in a 1954 photo, taken at a time when they and others thought the disease had been conquered.

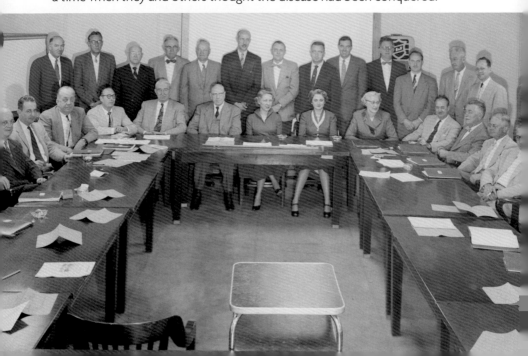

air. TB doesn't stay at home. It spreads through the air, and you get it by breathing. Diseases travel with people, and never has it been easier and faster to travel."[1]

Curing and even eliminating tuberculosis is not beyond the scientific capabilities of today, but it requires political will and the commitment of First World countries. TB experts say that millions of lives could be saved if the world's developed nations were to make eradication of TB a priority. The immediate effect would be felt in the world's poorest nations but ultimately all nations would benefit from such action.

More than fifty years ago the scientists who pioneered the first TB medicines thought they had made it possible to conquer tuberculosis. In the decades after the first cures, however, TB resurged, and the world must now fight a renewed battle against this old enemy. Says physician and TB expert Frank Ryan, "When, in the 50s and 60s, the pioneers placed the ball of tuberculosis eradication into our hands, we ran with it for a time and then we dropped it. The time has come to pick up the ball again, and this time we must run with it all the way to victory."[2]

CHAPTER ONE

What Is Tuberculosis?

Tuberculosis, or TB, is an infectious disease that has killed more people throughout history than any other disease, including bubonic plague, smallpox, or influenza. It is caused by a germ, a bacterium, which is difficult to kill and even harder to erase from human populations once it has gained a foothold. Tuberculosis is a complex and unpredictable disease. It can erupt into an active illness that causes severe disability and death, but the bacterium also can lie hidden within the human body for decades without doing harm. This inconsistent and erratic pattern makes it difficult to identify people who are infected and can pass the disease on to others. The pattern is even harder to discern because TB can attack so many different parts of the body. It may seem to take on the appearance of different diseases, and, indeed, tuberculosis once had many names.

For centuries doctors found TB almost incomprehensible. They would think a patient's disease was under control, only to see it roar back with strength and out-of-control virulence. They watched in puzzlement as tuberculosis spread wildly among some people yet seemed not to infect others. Some sickened people died within weeks, and others survived the disease for decades. Tuberculosis resisted the best medical efforts to understand it, treat it, or prevent it. Today, tuberculosis is well understood, but it is a disease that continues to surprise and challenge the medical world. It remains far from conquered, and to prevent epidemics requires worldwide dedication, unfailing medical vigilance, and multiple drugs.

Pulmonary Tuberculosis

The most common form of TB is pulmonary tuberculosis—a disease of the lungs. When left untreated it may follow a confusing and capricious course, but its outcome is easily predicted: It is usually a death sentence. When a person first becomes sick with tuberculosis, the symptoms may not look much different from flu, bronchitis, or a severe cold, but the symptoms signal something much more dangerous. Pulmonary TB usually starts with a cough and chest pains. Ryan says

A painter captures an 1823 piano performance by composer Frederic Chopin. Chopin later died of tuberculosis.

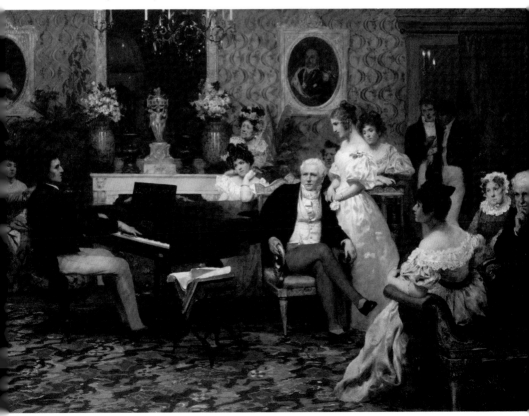

about the disease's victims, "They discover a cough which re-
fuses to go away; perhaps there is a sudden agonizing pain on
breathing."[3] The pain is the result of fluid building up in the
pleura, the membrane that envelops the lung. As the disease
progresses, breathing becomes more difficult, and the sufferer
becomes more and more exhausted. Then, sputum is coughed
up from deep within the lungs, as the lungs struggle to get rid
of the infection but fail. Sputum is a combination of pus,
phlegm, and bacteria. Eventually, blood is coughed up from
the lungs, as well. Blood in the sputum is from blood vessels in
the lungs that are being attacked by TB bacteria.

Other tuberculosis symptoms include fever that spikes
every evening, loss of appetite, a general wasting away of the
body, and night sweats. Usually, people sick with TB gradually
become more tired, more malnourished, and less able to
breathe as they slowly become bedridden. Conversely, the disease can sometimes progress very rapidly. No matter what the
speed of the disease, patients inevitably get weaker and
weaker. This apparent fading away is responsible for pulmonary TB's historical name—consumption. Lives and bodies
seem *consumed* by the disease.

Destructive and Deadly

All the consuming symptoms of pulmonary TB are the result
of bacteria that have attacked and ravished the lungs. Lungs of
people sickened with pulmonary tuberculosis are slowly destroyed as the bacteria eat holes in the lung tissue. Eventually
the victim dies a quiet death, if he or she is lucky. In some cases
the bacteria eat a hole in a major blood vessel in the body.
"When this happens," says Ryan, "the bleeding may be so tor-
rential that the victim dies from exsanguination, or from
drowning in his own blood."[4] Such an event is dramatic, but
death is only seconds away.

The inexorable march of tuberculosis meant an almost certain death sentence for people sickened with TB until well into
the twentieth century. No one knew, however, who would last
for years and who would be dead within weeks or months. TB
is unpredictable. At times people seem to recover and feel better,

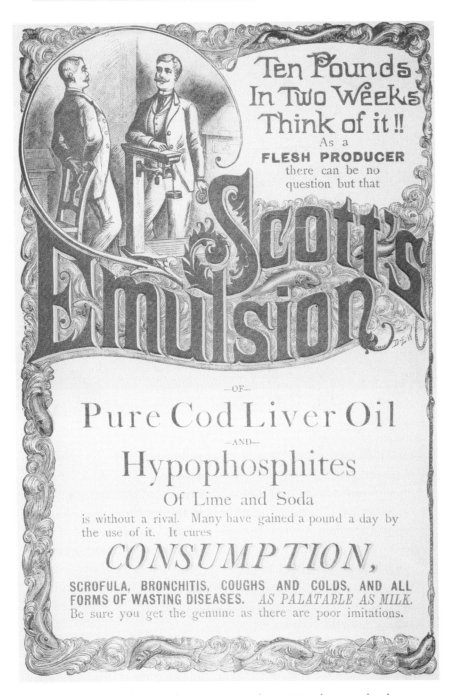

A cure-all advertised to desperate people in 1900 claims to heal tuberculosis, or consumption, as TB was once known.

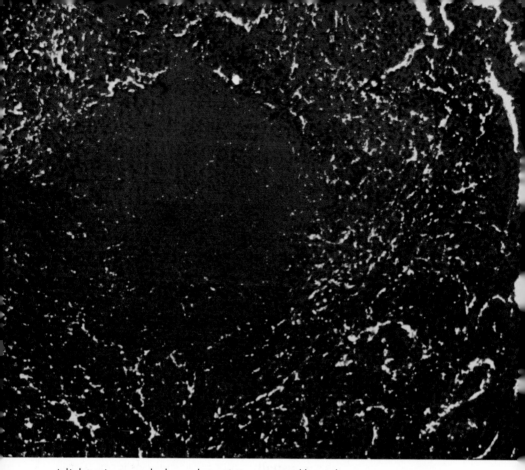

A light micrograph shows lung tissue ravaged by pulmonary tuberculosis.

but the improvement is almost always temporary. Eventually, even if it takes years, untreated patients succumb to the ravages of pulmonary tuberculosis. Because of this, people diagnosed with TB knew the shock of facing their own deaths when treatments were not an option. When the poet John Keats first saw the blood in the sputum he coughed up from his lungs, he said to a friend, "I know the colour of that blood—it is arterial blood—I cannot be deceived in that colour; that drop of blood is my death warrant. I must die."[5] A year later, in 1821, he did die of the disease.

Even in modern times the lungs of people who are untreated or who neglect their pulmonary tuberculosis show the destructive power of TB. Reichman describes the lungs of just such a patient with TB: "A healthy lung looks like a lively pink sponge," Reichman explains, but tuberculosis bacteria had eaten one lung in this victim until it looked like "a shrunken, ragged, shapeless piece of dark red tissue, almost like a piece of liver."[6]

Tuberculosis in Other Organs

Pulmonary tuberculosis is a terrible disease, but it is not the only kind of tuberculosis that tuberculosis bacteria can cause. TB germs can attack so many different parts of the human body that for centuries doctors believed they were dealing with separate diseases. This so-called "extrapulmonary" tuberculosis accounts for about 25 percent of TB infections today, but in the past, probably because people were less healthy, it was more common. TB can attack brains, bones, skin, the glands in the neck called lymph nodes, and almost any other body organ. One particularly severe form of TB is called miliary tuberculosis. In miliary TB the tuberculosis bacteria escape the lungs and travel in the bloodstream throughout the body. In this form tuberculosis can attack any organ in the body and destroy it. Ryan calls this form of the disease "one of the most lethal complications of tuberculosis."[7] Another form, tubercular meningitis, usually attacks infants and young children. In this manifestation of TB, bacteria invade the meninges, which are the coatings of the brain and spinal cord. Coma and death can quickly follow.

TB can also enter the bones and eat holes in them, just as it eats the lungs in pulmonary tuberculosis. During the nineteenth and early twentieth centuries this form of TB occurred commonly in children. Physician and medical historian Stanley B. Burns says, "The infection, as it dissolved joints and bones, contorted the limbs. The condition progressed until the joint or bone was no longer recognizable. When the infection broke through the skin, the joints and infected bones became riddled with holes, draining tuberculin pus. The pus helped to spread the disease . . . which often proved fatal."[8] When TB germs get into the lymph glands, the glands in the neck swell horribly; ulcers form on the skin of the neck and face, break open, and discharge pus; the fever, chills, and weight loss of pulmonary TB debilitate the victim; and when untreated this

TB can also lead to death. In the past this kind of tuberculosis was named scrofula and was not even recognized as a form of tuberculosis. As Ryan concludes, "Tuberculosis has the capacity to infect every internal organ, from liver to brain, from the fingertips to the delicate structures of our eyes."[9]

Miliary TB

Miliary tuberculosis is TB that has disseminated, or spread, throughout an organ or the body by means of the bloodstream. The affected tissues are dotted with tiny wounds called lesions that can be seen by X-ray or under a microscope. To the scientists who discovered them, these lesions looked like grains of millet. So this form of TB was named "miliary" after millet seeds.

A colored lung X-ray exhibits the many small lesions characteristic of miliary TB.

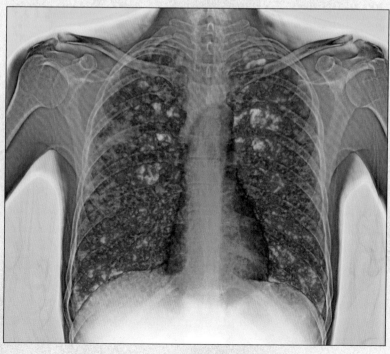

Latent TB

As horrifying and deadly as tuberculosis can be, however, the amazing thing about TB bacteria is that they usually do not make an infected person sick at all or may not make a victim ill until decades after he or she has been infected. A person can have TB and still not be sickened by it. All of the ways that TB kills are the result only of active tuberculosis. About 10 percent of infections with the tuberculosis bacteria become active and sicken the victim. The other 90 percent of the time, a person who has been infected with TB bacteria has no symptoms. This is called latent tuberculosis. The bacteria remain alive in the person's body, but seemingly do no harm. Such a person remains perfectly healthy. Even an untreated person with active tuberculosis, while not cured, may seem so when symptoms disappear, and the bacteria and the disease become latent.

The bacteria that cause tuberculosis are odd and behave in variable ways, unlike bacteria that cause other diseases. Why latent tuberculosis becomes active tuberculosis is sometimes still mysterious, but scientists and doctors understand how the process takes place and what makes it more likely to happen. The secret of TB's success as an invader and its ability to hide in the human body lies in the special properties of the bacterium itself.

The Unique Germ

The bacterium that causes TB is called *Mycobacterium tuberculosis.* It is a living organism of microscopic size but fairly large in comparison to other bacteria. It is shaped like a slender rod, or bacillus, and protected by a hard, waxy coating or shell. The rod is about two to four micrometers long. (A micrometer is a thousandth of a millimeter, which is equivalent to .04 inches.) Although the bacterium dies in a few hours when exposed to sunlight, it can easily survive for months in dark dusty corners, or cracks in house floorboards, or in the well-oxygenated environment of a human lung.

Mycobacterium tuberculosis most often enters its human host by being breathed in from the air. Commonly, the air has been contaminated by the cough of someone who has active

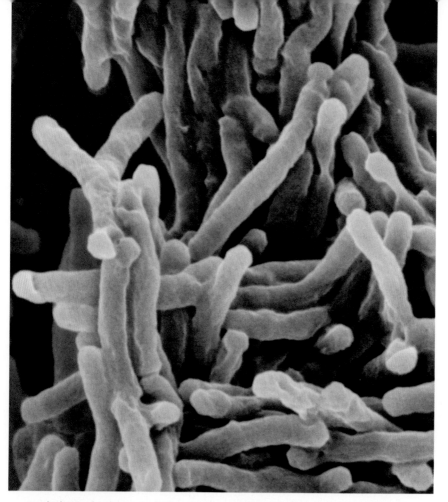

Rod-shaped tuberculosis bacteria are able to hide in the human body, sometimes for decades.

tuberculosis. That cough sprays water droplets that contain millions of living TB bacteria into the air. The water droplets evaporate quickly, but the bacteria can hang around in the air for hours. Spitting by a person with active TB releases bacteria into the air, too. Anyone who breathes this air may also breathe in *Mycobacterium tuberculosis*.

Body vs. Bacteria

Still, it is not easy for the bacterium to get into a person's lungs. The human body's defenses successfully fight off invasion in many cases. Bacteria can be caught by tiny hairlike cells that line the airway and either trap or expel the bacteria through the nose. They can be swallowed and destroyed by acids in the stomach. A few bacteria, however, may make it all the way down to a lung. Then, as Ryan explains, "What happens is basically simple if dreadful. The bacteria inhaled in water droplets settle in the periphery [outer edge] of the lung and grow very slowly until they form a small local collection, like a cheesy boil. From this boil, the continuing infection spills over into nearby small airways and forms more of these tiny boils."[10] These boils are called tubercles.

Again, human body defense systems come to the rescue, and often these defenses successfully contain the disease. When TB bacteria are detected by the body's immune system, infection fighters called macrophages rush in to attack the foreign invaders. Macrophages are white blood cells that swallow, eat

One Is Enough

Most bacteria reproduce or multiply by a process called binary fission. This means that no mate is necessary for a bacterium to reproduce. If a single bacterium is healthy and living in a good environment, it grows slightly larger. The DNA replicates, or copies itself, and each complete DNA strand attaches to opposite sides of the cell wall. Then the whole bacterium divides down its middle, as a new cell wall grows in its center. Once the cell wall is complete, the bacterium has now formed two identical daughter cells. Each of these daughter cells also can replicate itself by fission, or splitting into two. In many bacterial species, this process can occur again within twenty minutes after the daughter cells have formed. This means that a colony of bacteria could double in size every twenty minutes. Given enough food, one bacterium could become more than 1 billion in less than ten hours. This only occurs in the laboratory, however, since bacteria never have that much food available naturally. *Mycobacterium tuberculosis* reproduces much more slowly than other bacteria. Nevertheless, it follows the same process, and given time, it is capable of becoming huge colonies of millions of bacteria.

up, and destroy bacteria, but because of *Mycobacterium tuberculosis*'s hard, waxy shell, this job is not easy. The only time TB bacteria are vulnerable is when they are dividing in two in order to reproduce. Unlike other bacteria, though, TB bacteria divide extremely slowly—only once every twenty-four hours instead of the normal once every twenty minutes. The macrophages are thwarted in their attack, and the bacteria fight back, sometimes killing the macrophages instead.

It is as if a war is taking place inside the infected person's lung. Reichman describes the next stage of the war this way: "More macrophages rush in to stem the invasion. The TB bacteria, like the opportunistic parasites they are, break into the macrophages and begin multiplying inside them. Then they burst out through the walls of the helpless and spent defense cells. Desperately, other macrophages rush in and gobble up the debris [the dead cells], only to be commandeered by the TB bacteria."[11] This is how tubercles grow in the human lung. Often, in the end, the macrophages win, usually in about three or four weeks. The bacteria are not killed, but they are walled off by the body in a hard shell or membrane that contains them and prevents them from spreading further. When this happens, the person has latent tuberculosis. The TB bacteria are still in the lung but inactive and unable to spread. For most people, this is the end of the story. They stay healthy for the rest of their lives.

Lying in Wait

Still, for about 10 percent of people with latent TB, the war is not over. Decades may pass as the bacteria hibernate, alive and waiting. Then, perhaps when the body's defenses are weak— from another disease or from malnutrition, for example—the bacteria break out of their prison. This is when they multiply rapidly, eat holes in lungs, and travel throughout the bloodstream. The sputum that is coughed up by a person with active TB is a mixture of pus, destroyed macrophages, TB bacteria, and phlegm. In a person who is already weak with hunger or sickness or just infancy or old age, the bacteria may break out within days of the initial battle. These people also are on a path to death.

Tuberculosis Strikes

When a person with active TB coughs or sneezes—spraying millions of *Mycobacterium tuberculosis* into the air—a person who breathes in the contaminated air may become infected with the disease.

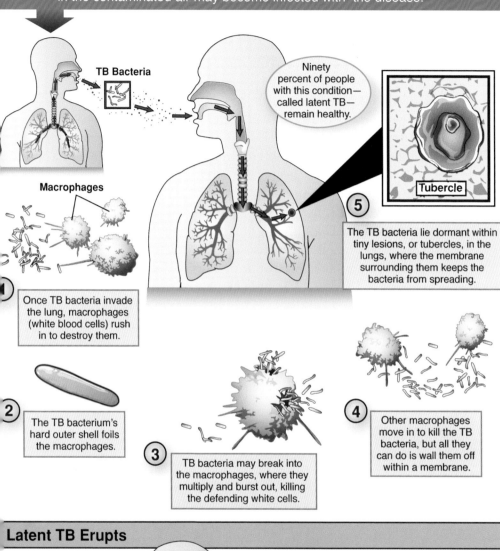

TB Bacteria

Ninety percent of people with this condition—called latent TB—remain healthy.

Tubercle

Macrophages

(5) The TB bacteria lie dormant within tiny lesions, or tubercles, in the lungs, where the membrane surrounding them keeps the bacteria from spreading.

(1) Once TB bacteria invade the lung, macrophages (white blood cells) rush in to destroy them.

(2) The TB bacterium's hard outer shell foils the macrophages.

(3) TB bacteria may break into the macrophages, where they multiply and burst out, killing the defending white cells.

(4) Other macrophages move in to kill the TB bacteria, but all they can do is wall them off within a membrane.

Latent TB Erupts

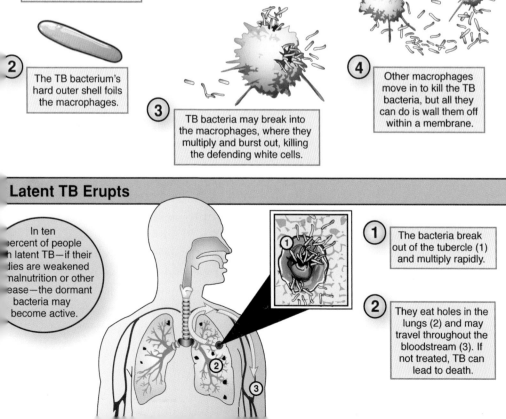

In ten percent of people with latent TB—if their bodies are weakened by malnutrition or other disease—the dormant bacteria may become active.

(1) The bacteria break out of the tubercle (1) and multiply rapidly.

(2) They eat holes in the lungs (2) and may travel throughout the bloodstream (3). If not treated, TB can lead to death.

Stealthy Bacteria

So, because of the unusual bacteria that cause TB, predicting its course or even knowing when a person is infected or at risk can be extremely difficult. This slow-growing, sometimes-winning, sometimes-losing bacterium spent centuries confusing doctors, mystifying cultures, and hiding its true origins. People with active tuberculosis coughed, laughed, talked, breathed, and spit, sending TB bacteria into the air around them and often infecting their children, their neighbors, and their caretakers. The disease was passed from person to person, but not quickly enough or predictably enough for societies to recognize how it was spread. Not until science advanced enough to identify the bacterium and develop treatments for it was tuberculosis possible to bring under control.

Even today, a tuberculosis outbreak may infect many people before it is discovered. People may be exposed to TB frequently in some parts of the world, but if they are healthy and have strong immune systems, no harm is usually done. About a third of the world population has latent TB. These people cannot spread TB to others. They do not shed tuberculosis bacteria in their coughs or spit. Only when body defenses break down and active TB emerges are they a threat to others. Even then, the people who are exposed and infected may develop only latent TB. When an outbreak of active TB occurs, it usually occurs in conditions of poverty.

Taking Advantage of Weakness

Poverty and tuberculosis are inextricably linked. Poor people often live in dark slum shelters and houses that lack fresh air and sunlight. Their diets often consist of foods that have little nutritional value. They are commonly prey to sickness and disease and have poor access to medical care. Since sunlight kills TB bacteria quickly, dark homes are places where TB bacteria can survive. If regular cleaning and sanitation are not possible, tuberculosis bacteria, once released into the environment, can lie hidden in cracks and crevices for long periods. Bodies that are not fed properly have weakened defense systems that do not do a good job of fighting off invading bacteria. When

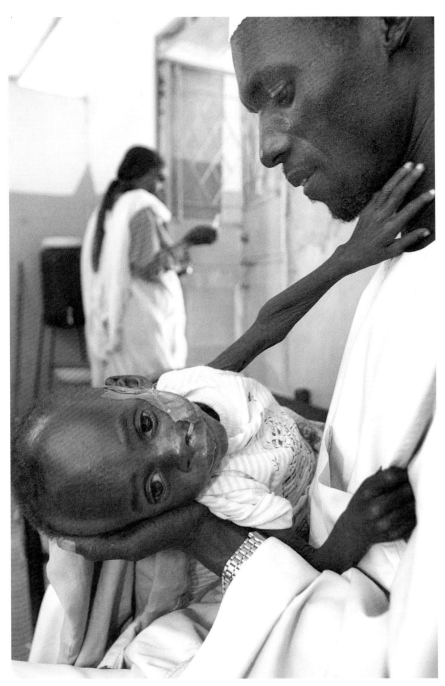

Poverty and tuberculosis often go hand in hand. Here a man from Sudan cradles his undernourished son, who suffers from TB.

immune systems are already battling other diseases, they are under stress. TB bacteria often win their war with the macrophages when immune systems are overwhelmed by stress and malnutrition, and active TB is the result.

Tuberculosis, however, is not just a disease of the poor. Once a TB outbreak has begun, it can spread anywhere. People of all social classes are exposed, and those with weakened immune systems may be at risk of active TB. Children and young people seem to be especially vulnerable, and yet it is almost impossible to avoid TB bacteria when the disease is already active in one part of the community. After all, people get TB just by breathing, and no one knows when the air may be contaminated. The airline travel and mobility of the modern world make an outbreak of TB highly possible in any area of the world.

Exposed and Infected

In a New Jersey hospital in the early 1990s, doctors got a good lesson in how TB infection can leap from one person to another. A young girl from Haiti named Merlande was being treated for tuberculosis that she had caught from her father in Haiti. The hospital kept Merlande isolated and provided her with a mask to help avoid spread of the bacteria. Visitors to Merlande's room were also required to wear masks. Merlande was far from home and family and very lonely. A medical student, Beth Malasky, visited with Merlande often and tried to cheer her up. Malasky said, "She was so sick she could barely stand, but when I came into the room, she'd be standing up in the crib looking through the bars like it was a cage."[12] Merlande loved the attention. She often tried to pull off her mask, but Malasky did not mind. She knew she was healthy, and Merlande was not coughing. Malasky played with Merlande and even hugged and kissed her.

The contact did not seem too dangerous, but soon Malasky was medically checked, and the tests showed that she had developed latent TB. So as not to risk developing active TB, she had to be treated with tuberculosis medicines. She remembers, "Eight pills a day. They were very large and hard to get down. I would gag when I tried to take them. The idea of not taking anything and hoping I wouldn't get sick was very appealing."[13] Malasky did complete her course of treatment, but if she had not had the medical knowledge of the danger, the TB spread might not have stopped with her. She could have developed active TB, breathed the bacteria on another person at the hospital or at home, who could have infected other people, perhaps on a bus or at a party, who would have spread the disease in an ever widening circle. The disease may start with one contact with a poverty-stricken child, but then it can move into any area of the population. This is how epidemics come into existence, and epidemics have always been the specialty of *Mycobacterium tuberculosis*.

CHAPTER TWO

Deadly Mystery

Epidemics do not always appear suddenly, kill thousands, and then disappear, such as flu epidemics do. An epidemic can also be an unexpected upsurge in cases of a disease that is already present in a community. Tuberculosis has followed this pattern for centuries. It has infected humans since at least eight thousand years ago, and until the bacterium was identified and medicines were developed, its cycle of epidemic remained irreversible. Scientific advances began to bring tuberculosis under control in the twentieth century, but before that time TB was a source of fear and dread throughout the world.

Since Ancient Times

Scientists have discovered TB in the bones of Egyptian mummies and of prehistoric cave people. Tuberculosis apparently infected societies independently in all parts of the globe. Since it was not carried from one group to another, many experts speculate that the disease originally began in cattle and was spread to people through cows' milk. Then the TB bacteria learned to live and grow within their human hosts. Even today, people can get TB by drinking unpasteurized milk from infected cows.

In the Western world, TB was described by the ancient Greeks who named it *phthisis*, from the Greek word for "wasting" or "decay." Hippocrates, the famous Greek physician, called TB the "almost always fatal disease of the lungs."[14] By the Middle Ages TB was spreading more and more in Europe. People were moving from isolated villages and farms into cities, where they lived crammed together in small rooms and often even shared beds. When people with active TB breathed bacteria into the air, the conditions were perfect for passing the disease to others, and these others had immune systems unable to fight off infection. Then the Industrial Revolution began, and things got worse.

The White Plague

The Industrial Revolution began in England, Ireland, and Scotland in the late seventeenth century. It was characterized by dark, crowded, unsanitary factories and mills. *Mycobacterium*

Scientists have found TB in the ancient bones of Egyptian mummies like this one photographed lying in its coffin.

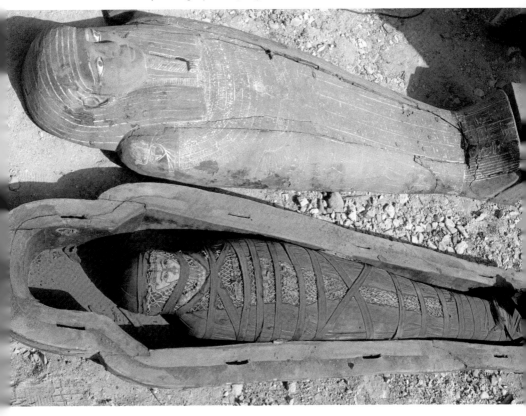

tuberculosis had perfect conditions in which to live, grow, and spread. Epidemics of tuberculosis exploded. The Industrial Revolution began a few decades later in the United States, but the conditions for the poor were the same as in Britain and Ireland, and TB was rampant in America, too. By the end of the nineteenth century, one in four people in Europe and in many industrial parts of the United States were infected with tuberculosis.

Western civilization was terrorized by tuberculosis which became known as the White Plague or the White Death in a graphic description of pale, wasted TB sufferers. Tuberculosis epidemics were even more frightening because no one knew what caused them or where they came from. Many medical people believed that TB was an inherited disease because it so often ran in families. Others believed TB reflected exposure to bad air or a bodily weakness resulting from unnatural lifestyles. Some suspected that TB was caused by a germ, just as other infectious diseases had turned out to be, but no one had ever been able to find such a germ in TB patients. Many doctors were certain that tuberculosis could never be treated or cured. They could offer diagnoses and drugs for pain but nothing else of value. Leeches often used in medicine during that time for ridding the body of "bad blood," for instance, just killed weakened TB patients more quickly.

The Culprit Unveiled

The first breakthrough in understanding tuberculosis came in 1882, when Robert Koch discovered the bacterium that causes TB. Koch was a country doctor in Germany who spent six years searching for the organism that could be proved to cause tuberculosis. *Mycobacterium tuberculosis* was so difficult to find because it was extremely difficult to stain. Without using stains to color bacteria, scientists could not see them under microscopes. The hard, waxy shells protecting TB bacteria were the problem. After much labor and creative experimenting, Koch solved the staining puzzle. More years were spent testing the bacterium to be sure it really was the cause of TB.

When Koch felt sure he had proof, he went to Berlin and reported his findings at a prestigious medical conference. He was

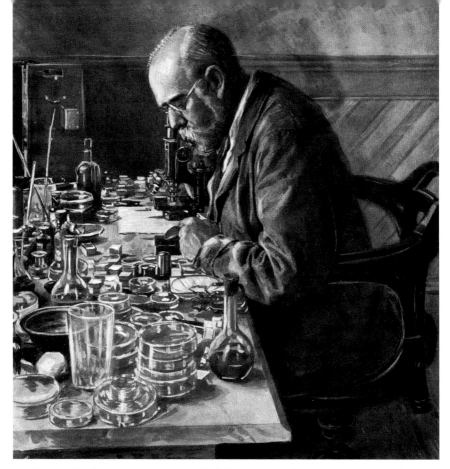

Pictured in his laboratory in an 1869 lithograph, German scientist Robert Koch is credited with discovering the bacterium that causes TB.

not sure if he would be believed. He began his report by reminding his fellow doctors how devastating TB was, and his statement reveals just how epidemic TB was at that time. Koch began,

> If the importance of a disease for mankind is measured by the number of fatalities it causes, then tuberculosis must be considered much more important than those most feared infectious diseases, plague, cholera and the like. One in seven of all human beings dies from tuberculosis. If one only considers the productive middle-age groups, tuberculosis carries away one-third, and often more.[15]

Koch went on to give a detailed demonstration of his discovery of *Mycobacterium tuberculosis*. As his audience sat in stunned silence, Koch explained that the bacteria he had found were always present in diseased organs. Furthermore, these bacteria could be grown in petri dishes in the laboratory. When they were injected in experimental animals, such as guinea pigs, they invariably caused the animal to develop tuberculosis. Koch finished, "All these facts taken together can lead to only one conclusion: that the bacilli [bacteria] which are present in the tuberculosis substances not only accompany the tu-

The hard outer capsule of *Mycobacterium tuberculosis* (pictured) stymied scientists in their attempts to treat TB.

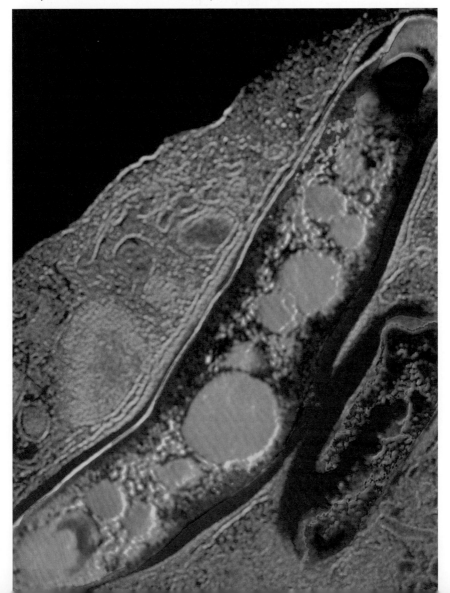

berculosis process, but are the cause of it. In the bacilli we have, therefore, the actual infective cause of tuberculosis."[16]

It was an amazing discovery, and the news traveled with lightning speed throughout the medical world. Although a few doctors refused to believe in the beginning, most were filled with hope that, for the first time, there was a possibility that TB could someday be cured. Said Paul Ehrlich, a prominent scientist who was in Koch's audience, "I hold that evening to be the most important experience of my scientific life."[17] Doctors and scientists everywhere began studying *Mycobacterium tuberculosis* in an excited search for the medicine that might halt the deadly disease.

Impossible to Crack

Unfortunately, their optimism was soon dashed. Despite their identification of the infectious bacterium, they could find no medical treatment that affected it. As late as the 1940s one medical professor of chest diseases claimed, "All work towards finding a chemical cure for tuberculosis is senseless because the bacteria are encapsulated in such a way that they are out of reach of such therapies."[18] It would be more than sixty years after Koch's groundbreaking presentation before scientists found an antibiotic that could break through that impervious shell. Medical efforts turned instead to prevention of TB's spread within the population and to helping victims' immune systems to fight the deadly bacteria.

Within a few years of Koch's discovery doctors did learn to isolate patients with TB from other hospital patients. In 1886 France passed the first law in the world against spitting in public places. This law was a reaction to a French scientist's discovery that the bacteria in sputum could be ground under a shoe and then dried out, rewet (as if rained on), dried again, wet again—up to eight times—and still live with enough strength to kill a guinea pig exposed to the sputum. In 1887 a hospital in London passed the first regulation that the spittoons in its wards had to be emptied and disinfected once a week. During the twentieth century clean, sterile hospitals and public education about the dangers of TB infection became the norm.

The Sanatorium Movement Begins

Tuberculosis epidemics slowed but did not disappear. In the end, it was impossible to prevent a disease that could be caught just by breathing at the wrong time. Doctors believed that they would never have a way to cure TB, but they were healers by profession. They desperately wanted to treat and offer hope to TB victims. In the United States, Edward Trudeau, a medical doctor and TB sufferer himself, became one of the leaders of a new rest therapy that provided tuberculosis victims with a healthy environment where their bodies might be able to fight TB naturally. He began the sanatorium movement in the United States: the establishment of institutions for TB victims where medical treatments of food, rest, and exercise were given to long-term patients.

Trudeau had cared for a brother who died of tuberculosis in 1865. He knew firsthand the horror and despair of a TB diagnosis. In 1873 he was told by his doctor that one of his lungs was riddled with TB and the other was beginning to be affected. Trudeau later remembered,

> I think I then knew something of the feelings of the man at the bar who is told that he is to be hanged on a given date, for in those days pulmonary consumption was considered an absolutely fatal disease. . . . And my rose-coloured dreams of achievement and professional success in New York, all lay shattered now; and in their place only exile and the inevitable end remained.[19]

Ill and dying, Trudeau decided to spend the last days of his life as happily as he could. He went into the wilderness, to Saranac Lake in New York's Adirondack Mountains, which he had loved since childhood. There he checked into an inn and spent months resting, fishing, walking in the fresh air, and eating simple healthy food. To his surprise he began to get better and gained weight. He reported, "Little by little, lying out under green trees and looking out onto water and the hills in tranquility, my fever subsided and my health—and with it my desire to live—began to return."[20] Trudeau felt that the healthy environment had given him miraculous new life.

Life in a Sanatorium

When Trudeau read of Koch's discovery of *Mycobacterium tuberculosis*, he did experiments of his own with rabbits and concluded that those in healthy environments got well, while those in dark cages died of their disease. He decided to build a sanatorium for TB patients at Saranac Lake where others could be healed as he thought he had been. During the twentieth century thousands of such sanatoria were established throughout Europe and the United States and became the standard treatment for tuberculosis patients. If patients were not cured, at least life was prolonged for many. TB patients typically spent two or three years at a sanatorium. They were prescribed extensive bed rest, rich full meals, milk every four hours, many hours of fresh air, gentle exercise, and carefully

A tuberculosis patient gazes out a window during her convalescence at Trudeau Sanatorium, built by sanatorium movement leader Edward Trudeau.

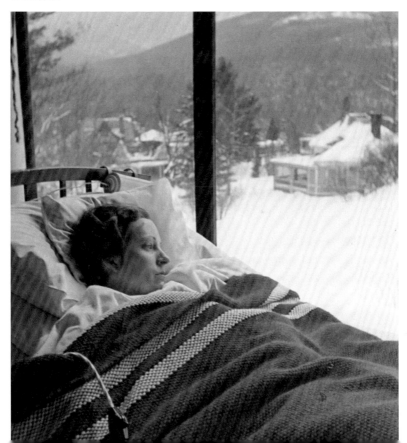

TB of the Rich and Famous

Throughout the Western world the number of famous people who died of TB is amazing. The authors Emily and Charlotte Brontë, for instance, both died of tuberculosis. Their brother Branwell and sister Anne succumbed to TB, too. Nineteenth-century writers who died of TB include Henry David Thoreau, Anton Chekhov, Fyodor Dostoyevsky, Franz Kafka, Katharine Mansfield, Robert Louis Stevenson, Edgar Allen Poe, and Stephen Crane. The composers Frederic Chopin and Wolfgang Amadeus Mozart were TB victims. Artist Amadeo Modigliani died of TB, as did actress Vivien Leigh. In 1962 Eleanor Roosevelt, wife of President Franklin D. Roosevelt, died of an old TB infection. Even the Old West gambler Doc Holliday died not in a gunfight, but of tuberculosis.

Film star Vivien Leigh, shown here with Clark Gable in a scene from *Gone with the Wind*, died of tuberculosis.

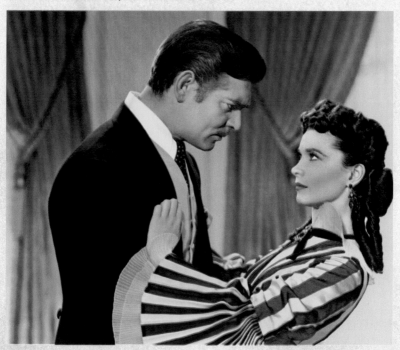

controlled lives. Rest was so important that some sanatoria did not even allow patients to feed themselves. They were carefully spoon-fed as they lay perfectly still in bed, forbidden to talk or laugh. Others were required to sleep outside, no matter what the weather, so as to be exposed to fresh air. The medical world had nothing else to offer.

Betty MacDonald, an American author, was diagnosed with tuberculosis in 1938 and spent a year in a sanatorium. In her journal she explains the rationale of the treatment:

> If you had a broken leg you wouldn't dance on it nor walk on it but would have a plaster cast or splints on it so that you couldn't use it even if you were foolish enough to try. If you had a sore on a joint or a knuckle, you would know that constant bending would break the sore open and prevent its healing quickly. When you have tuberculosis you have broken lungs with sores on them and the less you use them the quicker they will heal. How can you rest your lungs? By breathing less often and less deeply. A person resting quietly in bed, breathes two times less each minute than a person sitting up and of course much less than a person walking. . . . Rest is the answer. Rest, rest, and more rest.[21]

MacDonald did get better. Her active TB became latent, and she was eventually able to go home. Many patients in sanatoria improved, perhaps because their immune systems grew stronger, but many died of their disease either at the sanatorium or later, at home. Trudeau himself continued to have increasingly severe flare-ups of his active disease and eventually died of TB in 1916. There was never any proof that rest cures in sanatoria worked, but at least people with active tuberculosis were kept separated from the general population and did not pass the disease on to others.

"TB Blues"

Many people with active tuberculosis, however, refused to go to sanatoria. They were depressing places, where patients had little control of their daily lives, where deaths were common, and any meaningful, purposeful life was unattainable. These people simply continued their lives as best they could until the disease made activity impossible. One such TB sufferer was the country blues singer Jimmie Rodgers. He continued to travel America and perform his songs despite his debilitated condition and a body ravaged by TB. In a song he wrote in

Despite battling TB, country blues singer Jimmie Rodgers continued performing.

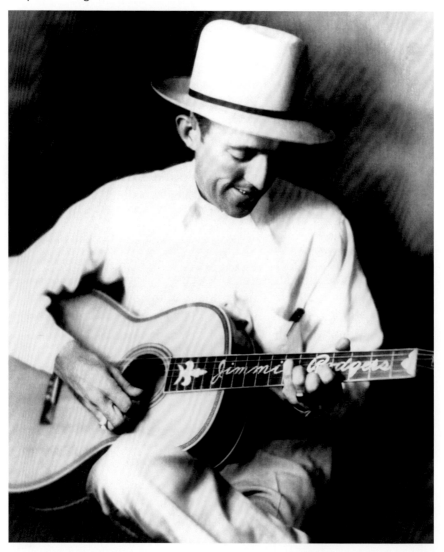

1931, "TB Blues," he sang of his failing battle, "I've got that old TB I can't eat a bite. Got me worried so I can't even sleep at night. . . . I've been fightin' like a lion looks like I'm going to lose. . . . I've got the TB blues."[22] He eloquently and honestly reflected the hopelessness of thousands of TB victims. Rodgers died of a lung hemorrhage in 1933.

The Breakthrough

Then, during the 1940s, what many believed to be impossible finally happened. Medical science discovered antibiotics—drugs derived from microscopic organisms that lived in the air or soil and had the capability of killing other microorganisms and bacteria. Most of these antibiotics, such as penicillin, were ineffective against *Mycobacterium tuberculosis*, but the antibiotic called streptomycin, which was discovered in the United States by Selman Waksman and Albert Schatz, was the longed-for miracle. In addition, unlike other chemicals from microorganisms, it did not poison people—only the TB bacteria in their bodies. It might cause uncomfortable or even disabling side effects, but the treatment would not kill the patient.

Schatz's scientific colleagues had warned him that searching for a medicine to cure TB was a waste of time. He remembered,

> They told me that the tubercle bacilli were covered with a heavy waxy capsule and nothing could get in. And that's why the drugs were not effective. My feeling was that if nothing got in we wouldn't have tuberculosis, because nutrients [to feed the living bacteria] would have to get in and waste products would have to get out. If food and waste products could get through, so could an antibiotic. So that argument did not hold water with me. I therefore kept on working.[23]

In 1943 Schatz and Waksman determined that streptomycin was able to break through the hard, waxy shells of TB bacteria and destroy them.

In the same year, Jorgen Lehmann in Sweden developed another drug, called para-aminosalicylic acid, or PAS, that was amazingly effective against TB bacteria. It was a derivative of simple aspirin that blocked the ability of the germ to take in oxygen. It, too, proved safe for people when Lehmann dosed himself with the drug and suffered no ill effects. Eight years later a third drug was added to the TB arsenal. It was called isoniazid. Suddenly, within the space of only a few years, tuberculosis became a treatable disease.

Cured!

The initial efforts to treat TB patients with streptomycin were stunning. The first, a woman identified only as Patricia, was dying of pulmonary TB in a sanatorium in Minnesota in 1944. She was twenty-two years old and weighed just seventy-five pounds. Patricia agreed to be the test case for streptomycin therapy because she had nothing to lose. She was dying. Streptomycin was expensive and very difficult to make in quantity. Over a period of six months Patricia was treated with injections of streptomycin. The treatment was interrupted whenever the medicine supply ran out but would start up again as more streptomycin was made. Despite the problems, Patricia responded and got well. The director of the sanatorium exulted, "It was a story book ending. The patient made a remarkable recovery. She led a very active life. After leaving the sanatorium, she married and became the mother of three fine children."[24]

PAS was equally successful in Europe. It, too, was very difficult to manufacture, and the slow production meant that few people were treated with it in the early years. One of the first patients was a former soldier and medical student named Ake Hanngren, who contracted TB in one lung. He later wrote, "In 1946 it spread to my other lung too and soon it also involved my intestines and my throat. I was just a skeleton, lying in a hospital in Stockholm."[25] From the hospital, Hanngren was sent to a sanatorium, essentially to die. There he learned of Lehmann's discovery and wrote to him to beg for some of the new medicine.

Lehmann sent Hanngren a supply of PAS. Not even the sanatorium doctors knew about it. The first sign that it was working was that Hanngren's fever was lower, and he felt well enough to sit up in bed. Hanngren described what happened

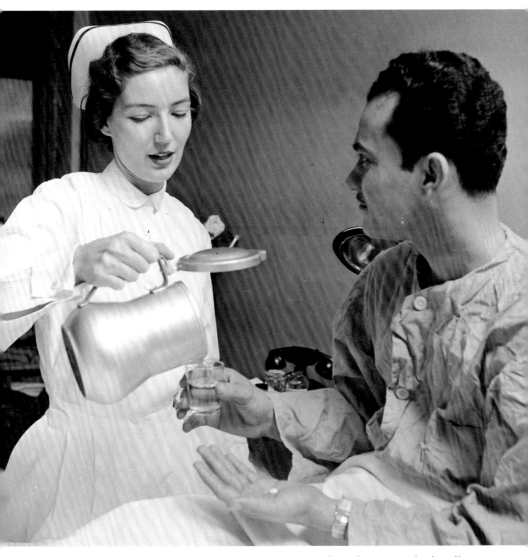

In this 1956 photo, a TB patient receives oral medication, which will be supplemented with injections of the potent drug streptomycin.

next: "After only one week or so, I could use the toilet in the corridor. I had been placed in a cubicle because I was dying. Now people could see me in the corridor. They realized that some miracle had happened. The physician was surrounded in his room by patients clamouring for the new treatment. He had to telegram Lehmann and after about six months he managed to get some PAS for his other patients.

"But I was healed. I recovered with no other therapy."[26]

Putting It All Together

PAS and streptomycin seemed almost like magic, but that magic often came with a price. Both were uncomfortable to take and caused side effects such as nausea, stomach pain, and even nerve damage. Some people were made permanently deaf. Others, such as the writer George Orwell, were so allergic that they had to be removed from treatment and subsequently died of their tuberculosis. Another strange problem was even worse. In many cases, patients' TB bacteria were not completely killed by either therapy. Patients seemed cured but then suffered relapses later and died of tuberculosis. It turned out that each drug killed most TB bacteria but not all. Some bacteria were resistant to the drugs. All TB bacteria were slow to die out completely, even under the best circumstances. By the 1950s doctors began to realize that TB treatment required a multidrug approach with long courses of treatment. They discovered that, slowly, what streptomycin did not kill, PAS could kill. What both PAS and streptomycin missed, the new drug, isoniazid, would catch. When patients were treated for many months with all three drugs combined, almost all were permanently cured of their disease.

In the 1960s other very powerful antituberculosis drugs were developed. Rifampicin, a derivative of streptomycin, was a stronger, safer medicine. Ethambutol replaced PAS. No bet-

Guns and TB

War, with its disruption of normal, healthy living conditions, creates ideal circumstances for the spread of tuberculosis. During World War II, for example, TB rates in Europe jumped dramatically. In Berlin, Germany, in 1937 (before the war) 77 out of every 100,000 people died of TB. By 1944 (late in the war) 225 of every 100,000 people were dying of tuberculosis. In Warsaw, Poland, in the same year, malnutrition was so widespread that 500 people out of each 100,000 died of TB.

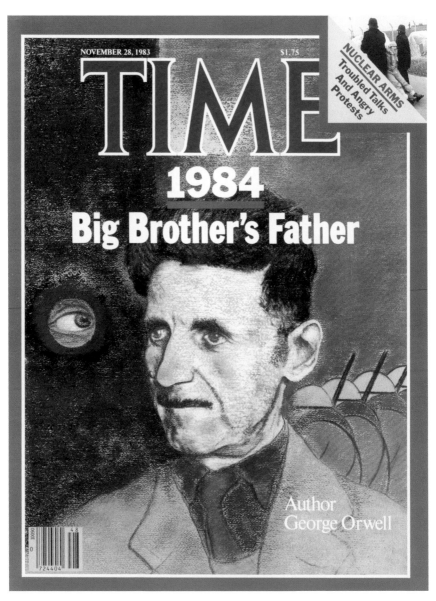

NOVEMBER 28, 1983 $1.75

TIME

1984
Big Brother's Father

NUCLEAR ARMS
Troubled Talks
And Angry
Protests

Author
George Orwell

Severely allergic to TB drugs, noted author George Orwell (in an artist's depiction on a *Time* magazine cover) had to discontinue treatment and died of the disease.

ter drug than isoniazid could be found, but pyrazinamide proved to be just as powerful. Other drugs were manufactured that were sometimes useful against the drug-resistant bacteria that were hard to kill. "Triple drug therapy," whether with the three original drugs or more modern mixtures, was stunningly effective at saving lives and preventing drug-resistant bacteria from surviving. These drugs were referred to as first-line drugs; the others were second-line drugs that had more side effects and were less often used. Eventually, the medical arsenal consisted of about nine anti-TB drugs. Death rates from TB fell, and sanatoria closed. At least in the Western world, tuberculosis was no longer a killer. Doctors even began to talk about wiping out tuberculosis in a slow but steady advance as it was conquered in poorer countries.

Biding Its Time

By the 1970s the general public had all but forgotten about tuberculosis. It was no longer a disease to be feared but a quaint, outdated story in history. TB, however, had not truly disappeared. In the Third World, poverty, war, and lack of medical facilities kept *Mycobacterium tuberculosis* alive. People still died by the thousands in quiet epidemics that went mostly unnoticed in First World countries. All along, tuberculosis was alive and well and biding its time.

CHAPTER THREE

The Disease That Fought Back

In 1998 a Ukrainian immigrant named Nikolay walked into a medical clinic in a small town in Pennsylvania with a hacking cough and pain in his chest. He had flown to the United States just three days previously. Nikolay was diagnosed with active TB, and his doctor reported the case to the Pennsylvania Department of Health, as he was required to do. In the United States, public health experts make every effort to track down, test, and treat anyone who may have been exposed to active TB so that it cannot gain a foothold and start an epidemic. Chest X-rays, TB tests, and laboratory examinations of TB germs coughed up in sputum are used to contain any spread of the infectious disease and to cure every identified tuberculosis victim. Even when the germ is latent, American patients are usually treated to prevent any future outbreak.

While public health officials searched for the people who had been passengers on the same plane as Nikolay, lab scientists were testing the bacteria from Nikolay's lungs. It was a long, tedious process. TB bacteria are still as slow to grow in laboratory petri dishes as they were in Koch's time. The tests confirmed *Mycobacterium tuberculosis* in Nikolay's sputum, but his doctors needed to know more. They needed to be sure which of the available TB medicines would best kill Nikolay's TB bacteria. This meant that cultures had to be grown in the

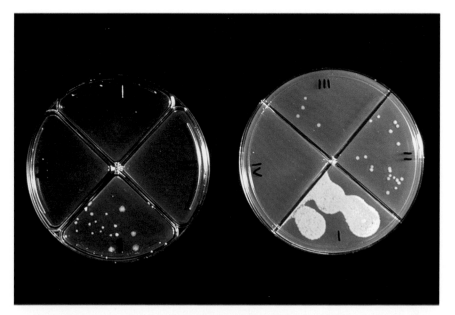

Growing in petri dishes, these laboratory cultures of TB bacteria are being tested for sensitivity to different drugs.

lab and tested for sensitivity with each different antibiotic. A dish where the germ kept growing when a drug was added was a dish with germs resistant to that medicine. After about a month Nikolay's results came back, and they were horrifying. Nikolay's TB bacteria were resistant to three first-line drugs—isoniazid, ethambutol, and pyrazinamide. Further testing revealed they were resistant to three second-line drugs as well. How could this have happened?

MDR-TB

Nikolay did not have ordinary tuberculosis, bad as that would be. He had a new, frightening kind of tuberculosis called multidrug-resistant tuberculosis (MDR-TB). In his native Ukraine, Nikolay had been treated three different times in the past for his tuberculosis. Each time, either because the drug treatment time had been too short or because the drugs were of poor quality, most of his TB bacteria had been killed, but not all. The resistant germs had multiplied and become stronger. By the time he reached the United States, Nikolay carried a particularly dangerous disease—one that was hard to cure and threatening to anyone who was exposed.

Testing for TB Exposure

In a failed attempt to develop a treatment for tuberculosis, Robert Koch discovered a way to tell if people had been exposed to TB infections. Whenever TB bacteria are detected by the body's immune system, antibodies are made to fight it. These antibodies stay in the body forever, ready to attack any new TB bacteria that invade. Koch killed TB bacteria and purified a liquid substance that could be injected into people sick with TB. It did not cure anyone, but it did cause a rash or welts to develop on the skin where the so-called tuberculin was injected. This happened because the body's antibodies recognized and attacked the dead bacteria. A modification of Koch's technique is used today to identify people with latent TB. A tuberculin skin test under the skin on an arm results in a localized reaction if a person has ever been exposed to TB. In First World countries, anyone with latent tuberculosis is then treated so that the disease will never become active.

A lab technician performs a tuberculin skin test.

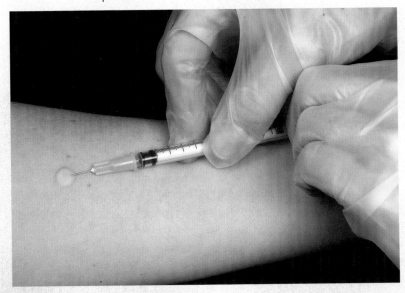

Luckily, Nikolay's MDR-TB could still be treated with rifampicin and streptomycin. Over a period of ten months he took these drugs daily and had his sputum tested over and over until it tested clear of TB bacteria. Then, just to be safe, he was treated for six months more. His wife, who tested positive for TB but had no symptoms, was treated as well. One of the public health officials involved in Nikolay's case was physician Bill Barry. Barry said, "Thank God he walked into the clinic in 3 days! He could have been in the community for 6 months, spreading tuberculosis that was resistant to six drugs."[27] As it was, no other people were identified as having caught the MDR-TB from Nikolay. In this case MDR-TB was caught and treated in time, but since its first appearance in the 1980s MDR-TB has terrified doctors and public health officials throughout the world.

TB's New Opportunity

Until 1985 cases of new TB infections in the United States had declined every year since TB drugs were discovered. Between 1985 and 1993 the incidence of TB rose by 14 percent. Partly, the increase was caused by political complacency. Tuberculosis seemed to be conquered. Public vigilance lapsed, and TB regained a foothold within the poor and weakened segments of society.

Pulmonary physician John F. Murray explains, "In an exercise of horrible judgment framed in the belief that the consistently declining rates of tuberculosis in the United States meant that the disease was no longer a threat—and over the dire predictions of public health experts—the U.S. Congress decided to save money by changing tactics." Instead of assigning a specific amount of money for tuberculosis control, between 1970 and 1972 Congress gave money to the states but left spending decisions up to them. States could spend the money as they wished. This meant that cash-strapped state governments spent less on TB programs. Murray notes that in New York City, particularly,

staffing and services shrank to their all-time low and outpatient clinics were cut from 24 to 8. This . . . dismantling occurred while the number of homeless was climbing; more and more people were turning to alcohol, heroin, and cocaine; mental institutions were shedding patients into the streets; and large numbers of immigrants from high-prevalence countries arrived laden with *M. tuberculosis.*[28]

Causes of MDR-TB

Homeless and substance-abusing people are often malnourished and have weakened immune systems. They and people from mental institutions tend to be poorly cared for and to seek medical care rarely. Immigrants joined the poor population, and, if they already had active TB, easily infected others around them. Many of these people did go to health clinics when they became sick, but that did not stop the problem. They were given appropriate treatment, and the necessity of a

Homeless people like this man are especially susceptible to TB, since they are often undernourished and may have weakened immune systems.

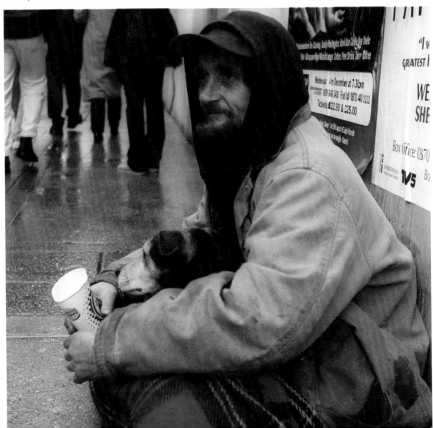

long course of medicine was explained to them. Many, however, stopped taking their medicines when they felt better. This caused some TB bacteria to die but others to survive and multiply. Health clinics did not have the funds to follow up on these patients and educate them on the importance of uninterrupted treatment. Just as Nikolay did, these people developed TB that was resistant to whatever drugs they had been taking. Little by little, because of incomplete treatment, this MDR-TB moved through parts of society.

In 1985, for example, a young woman from South Korea immigrated to the United States. She had active tuberculosis, and her treatment in her homeland had been interrupted. Doctors in America treated her with triple drug therapy for four months, but she only got worse. When her TB bacteria were tested, doctors discovered that the bacteria were resistant to seven antituberculosis drugs. In desperation, her doctors turned to the old-time drug, PAS, along with a few other second-line drugs. Eventually, they were able to cure the woman successfully, but the experience horrified TB experts. They wondered what they would do if such a terribly resistant tuberculosis bacterium spread through the population, and they worried that it was just a matter of time before a bacterium arose that was resistant to every available drug.

TB and AIDS

Doctors did not realize it, but a worse problem was coming. The increase in tuberculosis was linked with a new disease that reached America in 1976, although it was not immediately recognized as a new disease. It was AIDS, a deadly infection that attacks and decimates the immune system. The AIDS epidemic created a perfect environment for the resurgence of tuberculosis and the spread of MDR-TB. Weakened immune systems had little chance when confronted with exposure to tuberculosis bacteria.

The Weird TB

In 1981 a doctor at the New Jersey Medical School University Hospital, Reynard McDonald, confronted his first case of a par-

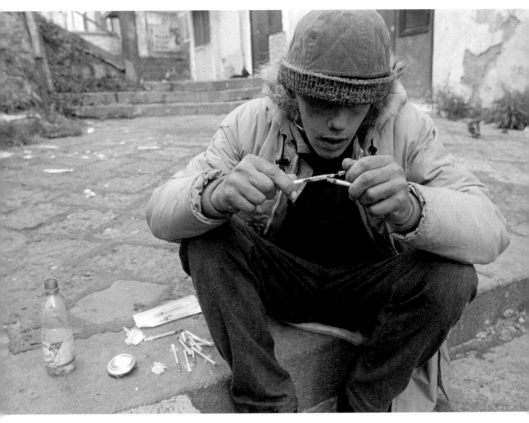

A drug user collects discarded needles. Reusing needles increases the likelihood of getting AIDS and other illnesses.

ticularly vicious and severe tuberculosis. The patient had pus-filled, inflamed areas in his brain caused by tuberculosis. These abscesses were causing brain tissues to disintegrate. McDonald was so concerned about this "weird TB" that he called in Reichman, his colleague, for a consultation. McDonald told Reichman, "I've never seen it before."[29] It would not be the last time, however, that the two tuberculosis experts would see this terrible TB. The sufferers were either gay young men or drug abusers who injected their drugs.

The doctors did not know at that time why these people had such weakened immune systems that caused the strange, virulent forms of TB. Reichman later remembered, "The first American cases of AIDS had been reported in 1981. . . . We had no idea then how serious this dreadful synergy between AIDS and TB would become." Reichman and McDonald collected the

Prisons Have Always Been Hot Spots

Crowded prisons have always been places where TB rages. By the late nineteenth century, for example, in England's Chatham Naval Prison, half of all the prisoners died of tuberculosis every year. In the United States no prisoner given a life sentence survived more than twelve years, usually because of TB. Seventy-five percent of the prison deaths in Massachusetts each year in the early 1900s were from tuberculosis.

Inmates pose for a photograph at an Illinois prison in 1900. Tuberculosis ran rampant in prisons during the early twentieth century.

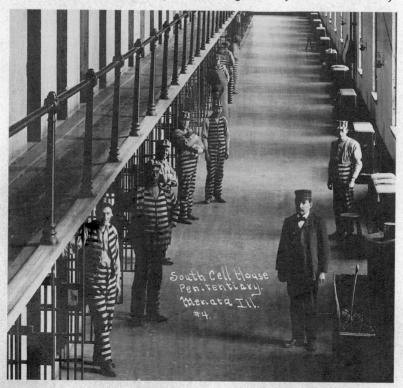

cases and reported on them in a medical journal in 1984. HIV, the virus that causes AIDS had not yet been identified, but the doctors could see what was happening. Explains Reichman, "People with normal immune systems usually have ordinary TB. But we reasoned that in a patient with a weakened immune system, TB might take on unfamiliar forms. Essentially, without a strong army of macrophages to contain the TB bacteria in the lungs, the infection is free to roam throughout the body."[30] This is just what was happening. HIV/AIDS was destroying immune systems. Tuberculosis bacteria invaded easily and multiplied wildly. Even worse, each disease helped the other to grow. As the AIDS epidemic spread, so did tuberculosis. By 1986 incidences of TB were increasing not only around New York City but in other areas in the United States and around the developed world.

The Renewed Killer

MDR-TB began appearing in the HIV/AIDS population. Some patients, such as drug users, were not completing courses of TB treatment medication and were developing and spreading a vicious TB that resisted TB drugs of choice. Then in 1991, in the *New York Times*, a newspaper headline appeared that shocked America: "A Drug-Resistant TB Results in 13 Deaths in New York Prisons."[31] Twelve prisoners and one prison guard had died of MDR-TB in the close, confined environment of the prison system. Eighty-four more prisoners were identified as exposed and had latent TB. Finally, the New York Health Department took the rise of tuberculosis and its drug-resistant strains seriously. The state began a concerted effort to find and eliminate the problem. The United States as a whole began an aggressive program to tackle tuberculosis and prevent a deadly epidemic. Public health departments determinedly worked to identify every case of active TB, treat each patient as long as required, and isolate patients where necessary to prevent exposing others. The vigilance paid off. By 1993 the crisis was over in the United States. TB cases began declining once again, but it was already too late to eliminate the problem completely. MDR-TB continued to show up in the most unexpected places.

In 1992 one of twin baby boys in an upper-middle-class New York community had a "cold" that would not go away. Only when his brother also became ill was the cold diagnosed as tuberculosis. Both parents and a sibling tested positive for the disease, too. The shocked mother said, "I felt so immune. We live in a tiny town in Westchester, in the middle of the forest."[32] No one ever figured out how the family had been exposed to TB, but this experience is repeated, here and there, in America and the rest of the developed world to this day.

A Complicated Equation

The resurgence of tuberculosis still frightens doctors who are knowledgeable about the White Plague, although TB specialists do understand the roots of the problem. Murray sums up, "The reasons for the resurgence are complex, but four factors have generally been implicated: the arrival and spread of HIV infection; immigration of people from high-prevalence countries; the development of 'hot spots' (e.g., hospitals, shelters, prisons) where tuberculosis flourished; and the deterioration of tuberculosis control."[33]

While an epidemic has been averted for now in the Western world, the multiple problems of MDR-TB, AIDS infections, poverty, and erratic treatment have not gone away. New cases of TB and deaths from TB infections continue to decline in the United States, as they do in most of the Western world, but tuberculosis has exploded in much of the Third World. There, doctors have little hope of containing the epidemic that is causing overwhelming suffering and millions of deaths and threatens to rage unchecked.

Prisons Are TB Hot Spots

Russia, not technically a Third World country but struggling to provide sophisticated medical services, is a TB hot spot. There, MDR-TB is a large, unsolved problem. Russia supports a vast prison system with almost a million prisoners. In these dark, airless, crowded institutions, people with tuberculosis are usually not separated from other inmates. They expose thousands of other prisoners to their TB bacteria. One prisoner said,

"When people arrive in prison they are all pushed into the collection room where nobody asks whether you have TB or not and people get infected from each other—it's unavoidable." Ill-clad and poorly fed, weakened and often sick, these prisoners rapidly progress to active tuberculosis infections. Another prisoner complained, "I know for certain that if I wasn't sent to prison then I wouldn't have caught TB. You are sitting in the same cell with many other people and you never know if someone has TB. TB is an additional punishment that shouldn't happen." Added a third prisoner, "We need to stop TB. If I'm guilty of a crime then punish me, but don't give me TB."[34] Prisoners in this system do receive medical care—if the medicine is available, if the hospital wards are not too full, if the doctor shows up, and if the prisoner is not released because his sentence was

A Moscow prison houses a tiny segment of Russia's huge prison population, which suffers from a high rate of MDR-TB.

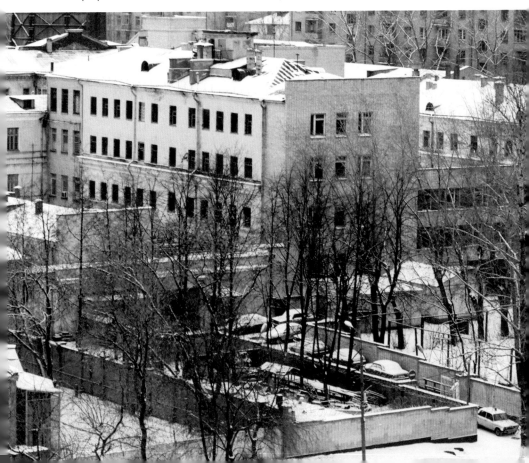

completed. Often, medicine is given for a little while and then stopped. Then it might start again, and then it stops. It is a perfect method for training TB bacteria to resist TB drugs.

Prisoners who are sent back to the community often do not receive any TB treatment. Multidrug-resistant TB has become common. It spreads to other prisoners and to prisoners' families, friends, and neighbors. A former Russian prisoner who tried to get medical care for his TB upon his release explains his situation this way:

> I was told that my medical records would be sent to the hospital, but they didn't get them. All I got from the prison was a reference of release. They were promising to make a passport [necessary for all Russian citizens], even took a photo, but I didn't get one. So, I will have to go around infecting people trying to get a passport because you have to have one.[35]

Few people can find or afford good medical care. Prisoners in Russia today have a TB incidence forty times higher than the rest of the population. About one in ten of all Russian prisoners have TB, and a tenth of those have MDR-TB. There is little money to upgrade prisons or for aggressive TB treatment plans in Russian communities.

But Not Confined to Prisons

The prison problem has inexorably spread to the general population. Physician Zulfira Kornilova, a dedicated Russian TB fighter, says, "There is now a group of patients who do not respond to any medicine. It is maybe 15 to 20 percent of all those who have MDR-TB." These patients almost invariably die, as do 40 to 60 percent of MDR-TB patients worldwide. Kornilova does the best she can, but since the fall of the Soviet Union in 1991, health care has badly deteriorated in Russia; she and doctors like her are often helpless. Kornilova would like to study and explore the super-MDR-TB in her country. "But there are no exact figures for the super-resistant forms," she says, "because the laboratories do not have the right equipment and are not clean enough."[36] Because of social and political conditions,

Russia has a full-blown epidemic of MDR-TB that is one of the worst in the world.

Sporadic medical treatment has caused the rise of MDR-TB in other developing areas, such as in South America and Asia. In many developing countries people can buy antibiotics over the counter without a doctor's prescription. People sick with TB buy and take drugs when they are ill, but they take these drugs only until they feel better. Tuberculosis bacteria gradually become resistant to these medicines. MDR-TB, however, is only one cause of the terrible, explosive resurgence of TB.

Africa's Scourge

Nowhere is the resurgence of TB as terrible as it is in Africa, an area of the world where few people ever have access to appropriate medical care. Especially in sub-Saharan Africa, AIDS is an explosive epidemic, and because of it, TB kills more people there than anywhere else on the earth. It is estimated that in 2004 about 14 million people worldwide had both HIV/AIDS and TB. Seventy percent of those people lived in sub-Saharan Africa. Ninety percent of untreated HIV-positive people with TB die within a few months, not of AIDS but of tuberculosis. Africa is not a hot spot for MDR-TB because few people in Africa are ever treated at all for their tuberculosis infections. Instead, they die of ordinary TB that is activated and spread by HIV/AIDS. Poverty, fear, and political disinterest contribute to the desperate situation and keep tuberculosis a plague that never stops.

In sub-Saharan Africa about 171 million people are infected with latent tuberculosis. According to history, only about 10 percent of these people should ever develop active TB, but exposure to AIDS changes this percentage drastically. As the AIDS epidemic in Africa grew out of control, an expert reported to the World Health Organization (WHO) in 1992, "Africa is lost."[37] Nothing contradicts that bleak prediction today. About half of the people with HIV develop tuberculosis, and the number of people with active TB grows by 10 percent every year. Swaziland, for instance, is a sub-Saharan country of about 1 million people. Almost 40 percent of the population has HIV,

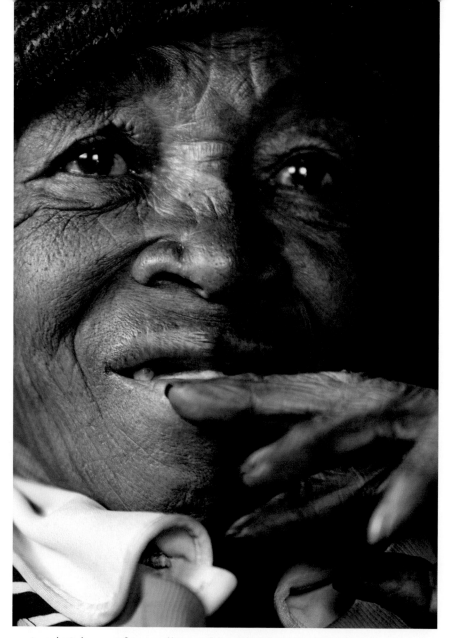

In sub-Saharan Africa, millions of people, including this woman, are afflicted with AIDS, which makes them more vulnerable to contracting TB.

and eighty-five out of one hundred thousand people in Swaziland die each year of TB. People with latent TB are eight hundred times more likely to develop active TB when they are infected with HIV. As a matter of fact, one-third of all deaths that are reported as being AIDS deaths are really TB deaths.

Tuberculosis, however, is not just a danger to AIDS patients. As pathologist and TB expert Thomas Dormandy explains, "AIDS-related tuberculosis did not mean that the upsurge in tuberculosis was confined to HIV-positive individuals: AIDS was merely the trigger for the new dissemination."[38] A person with active TB can infect, on the average, about ten to fifteen people each year if the disease is left untreated. In this age of easy global travel, ordinary TB, AIDS-related TB, and MDR-TB are dangers to every person on every single continent. Experts predict that a worldwide epidemic is inevitable unless something is done to stop the White Plague. Tuberculosis is a humanitarian crisis in the Third World, but it is also a threat to the entire developed world.

CHAPTER FOUR

Combating TB in the First World

Tuberculosis is rare in the United States today, and public health officials fight daily to keep it that way. In 2004 there were 14,511 reported cases of TB nationwide, and over half those cases were in newly arrived immigrants. Every diagnosed case in the United States is aggressively treated, and the cure rate is more than 80 percent. Because of the constant alertness of the U.S. Centers for Disease Control (CDC) and diligent medical treatment, the occurrence of MDR-TB has also been reduced dramatically. Only 114 people were reported to have MDR-TB in 2003, for instance. Most First World countries have seen similar declines in TB cases since the developed world increased its efforts to combat and control tuberculosis. In the United Kingdom, for example, most cases of TB also occur in immigrant populations, and only 0.1 percent of TB cases there are MDR-TB. This success means that few doctors ever see a case of active tuberculosis, but the success story no longer leads to complacency about the menace of TB and epidemics. The medical community is well aware that a lapse in vigilance could allow TB to roar back and threaten the health of every community. Every case of active TB is a warning that triggers a public health investigation, even when the individual patient is not in danger.

Cured, but Who Started It?

Usually a TB infection in the developed world is not a life-threatening event. A British man named Rupert, for instance, went to a London hospital because of a sore chest. He had worn a cast on a broken arm for several weeks and thought holding up the cast for so long had made his chest muscles ache. When doctors x-rayed his chest and diagnosed TB, Rupert almost thought it was a joke. The doctors were very serious, however, and Rupert found himself in an isolation room in the hospital where TB treatment was immediately begun. After a short time he was able to go home and continue his medication as an outpatient. Rupert remembers, "I worried about who might have infected me and whether I had infected anyone. . . . Even after a stay in the hospital, the road to complete recovery is a long one. If you are lucky, however, it is a straight road. All you have to do is take the pills and try to lead a relatively healthy life. I am happy to say that I had my share of luck and am now tuberculosis free."[39]

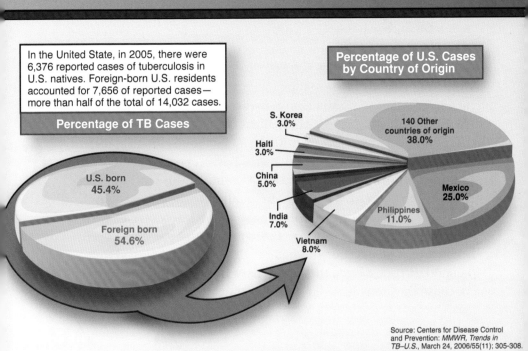

Reported Tuberculosis Cases in the United States by Country of Origin, 2005

In the United State, in 2005, there were 6,376 reported cases of tuberculosis in U.S. natives. Foreign-born U.S. residents accounted for 7,656 of reported cases—more than half of the total of 14,032 cases.

Percentage of TB Cases

U.S. born 45.4%

Foreign born 54.6%

Percentage of U.S. Cases by Country of Origin

S. Korea 3.0%
Haiti 3.0%
China 5.0%
India 7.0%
Vietnam 8.0%
Philippines 11.0%
Mexico 25.0%
140 Other countries of origin 38.0%

Source: Centers for Disease Control and Prevention: MMWR, Trends in TB–U.S., March 24, 2006/55(11); 305-308.

Drugs of Choice

Today, doctors have six first-line drugs for curing TB. They are isoniazid, rifampicin, streptomycin, ethambutol, thiacetazone, and pyrazinamide. The medicines are relatively cheap and effective against ordinary TB. Usually, four are used in combination for six to eight months in order to cure tuberculosis. In First World countries the cost to treat a patient is about $2,000. However, when a person has MDR-TB, the cost dramatically increases, both because treatment time is longer and because second-line drugs may have to be used. To cure a person with MDR-TB costs about $250,000 on average.

In 1998 another British patient, called Alexandria, experienced the same easy treatment course to a cure, but she also worried about how she may have become infected. Alexandria said, "I don't know how or when I contracted it (I'm told it could have been from traveling in third world countries, from being born in New York, from sitting next to someone on the bus or it may have lain dormant since my childhood and chosen 1998 to reveal itself)."[40]

Finding the Index Case

Although not always possible, discovery of the TB index case is a major goal of public health investigations when a patient with TB is diagnosed. Good medical detectives prevent many TB outbreaks in the First World. An index case is the first identified case of active TB. When such a person is diagnosed, U.S. doctors report the case to the CDC and to the state public health department. Then, public health workers search out anyone they can find who may have come into contact with the index case and encourage these people to be tested for TB exposure. The people who have caught TB are referred to as secondary cases. Even those who have no symptoms are tested because they may have latent TB. If they do, they are given TB treatments to cure their tuberculosis and prevent future active and infectious TB.

Reichman describes an example of one public health investigation in 1995 when an outbreak was discovered in rural communities in Kentucky and Tennessee. The first clue was a little girl who tested positive for TB exposure during a regular checkup at school. The child had latent tuberculosis and was not infectious, so she could not have been the index case. Public health officials checked all the members of the little girl's family and found an uncle, identified as "Charlie," who had active TB. He was the index case, and he had walked around for six months unknowingly infecting other people. Charlie had gone to his doctor when he first noticed a cough and chest pain, but the doctor had misdiagnosed Charlie with pneumonia. The antibiotics the doctor prescribed for Charlie had no

In Asia, a doctor in East Timor examines a man exhibiting TB symptoms.

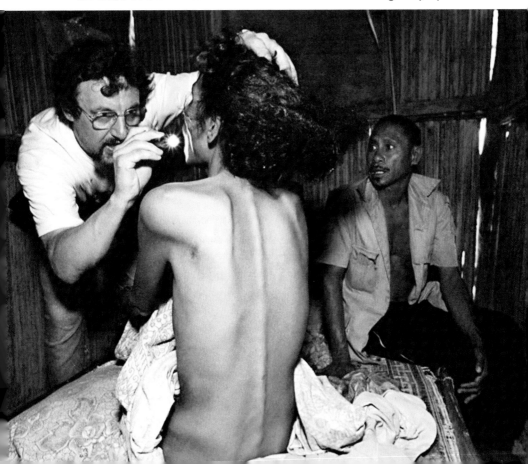

effect on his TB. Charlie felt worse and worse, but he continued to go to his job at a garment factory and to interact with his extended family. Unfortunately, as Reichman explains, "Charlie's TB was also unusually good at infecting people."[41]

Every one of Charlie's family members and close friends tested positive for exposure to TB. Five of those people developed active tuberculosis. Several of the people who worked at Charlie's garment factory also had latent TB. Two people who had once waited in the doctor's waiting room with Charlie developed TB. Half of the people on the doctor's staff were positive for TB exposure. Some friends who had hung out one night at a gas station with Charlie tested positive for TB. Luckily, all of these people, including Charlie, could be treated with first-line drugs and cured of their infections. The outbreak was stopped.

Despite a careful and thorough search, however, CDC workers were never able to determine who had infected Charlie. The CDC searched hospital records for every TB case in the two states but none were the same strain of tuberculosis bacteria that infected Charlie and his community. Where Charlie caught his TB remains a mystery. All the CDC workers were finally able to determine was that the outbreak had been stopped when all the secondary cases with Charlie's TB strain were finally identified and treated.

The Killer's Fingerprint

Tracing secondary cases from an index case is a major tool used by public health officials to prevent TB bacteria from gaining a foothold in society. It is one way that they know where an outbreak of tuberculosis has traveled and whether an index case is the only case that needs to be investigated. No one had to figure out, for example, all the people that the men at the gas station had been in contact with because the CDC knew that those men had caught their TB from Charlie. Theirs were secondary cases. Public health officials were able to identify the index case, the secondary cases, and Charlie's TB strain in the same way that police departments often find human killers. They used DNA fingerprinting, but the DNA fingerprint was not a person's fingerprint; it was the fingerprint of a tuberculosis bacterium.

DNA is the genetic material in every living thing that determines how it grows and functions. Within the cells of living things are coils and spirals of DNA that contain a code, like the letters in a giant book, that determines the characteristics of the organism. Even a one-celled organism such as *Mycobacterium tuberculosis* contains DNA, and this DNA varies from TB strain to TB strain, just as it varies from person to person in human beings. When *Mycobacterium tuberculosis* divides in order to reproduce, it must replicate its DNA, and sometimes variations, mistakes, or mutations occur during this copying process. These alterations will then be copied in all the proliferating bacteria of a particular strain. If they help the bacteria to survive and grow stronger, a successful strain is born. This is how particularly infectious strains, such as the one that infected Charlie, develop, and it is also how MDR-TB came into existence. Each strain has some genetic variation particular to it, and DNA specialists can determine that strain by identifying the genetic markers it carries. Most strains have been given letter names. The New York City Health Department, for example, has a computerized database that identifies and labels more than twelve thousand strains of tuberculosis bacteria from around the world. The W family is the most common TB strain in the United States, but variations of it—W1, W2, W3, and so on—exist with very minor differences. Scientists believe that the W family of *Mycobacterium tuberculosis* may have originated in Asia.

Making DNA Matches

The DNA fingerprint of a TB strain not only helps public health workers to identify secondary cases, it also is extremely valuable as a medical tool. If a previously identified strain is found in a TB patient, doctors also know from experience what kind of medicines will work best to kill it. In 2000 in New York City, for instance, Barry Kreiswirth of the Public Health Research Institute was asked to test a sputum sample from a hospitalized TB patient. Kreiswirth was able to identify the strain

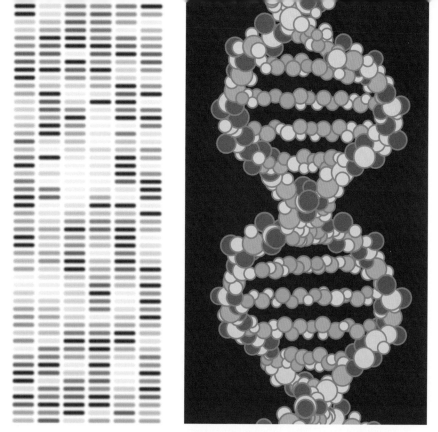

Shown here is a representation of a segment of a DNA molecule (right) and a laboratory printout of its DNA fingerprint (left). DNA encodes the genetic information for every living thing, including TB bacteria.

exactly because he had already received and identified TB samples of the strain. His samples are brought to him from around the world in small, sturdy cardboard boxes that are carefully sealed. The TB bacteria are killed by heat so they are no longer dangerous, and the DNA is extracted. "It's a powder," Kreiswirth explains. "It looks like dried snot."[42]

When the powder is analyzed and its fingerprint is determined, Kreiswirth and his team have a sample that can be matched to any other sample that they receive in their lab. This is just what they did with the sample from the New York City patient. The computerized database found a match. The patient's TB was the W148 strain, a strain that was already in Kreiswirth's database as MDR-TB that originated from a prison in Tomsk, Russia. Now Kreiswirth knew that the patient was probably a Russian immigrant and that he had MDR-TB.

Kreiswirth also knew that W148 is resistant to all four first-line TB drugs. He informed the hospital personnel who then knew which TB drugs to use in their patient's case.

Once, DNA fingerprinting not only identified a cluster of secondary cases of TB, it helped solve a crime. In 1999 there was an outbreak of TB in northern Florida. Over a period of fourteen months, thirty people were diagnosed with tuberculosis. The Florida Department of Health discovered that twenty-one of these people were infected with TB bacteria with identical DNA fingerprints. When the health workers searched for the mutual contacts of these victims, they discovered people running an illegal gambling and drug-trafficking operation who were the source of the infection. The state contained the TB outbreak and stopped a criminal activity.

Protecting Public Health

In the developed world DNA fingerprinting of *Mycobacterium tuberculosis* and public health investigations of TB outbreaks help to keep the chance of an epidemic very small. Proper medical treatment for the right amount of time for each and every identified patient is critical, too. TB's spread is prevented by positively ensuring that each person who has TB is treated until the infection is completely cured. Even more important, MDR-TB cannot develop when tuberculosis infections are treated correctly. Ordinary TB strains can be cured with a course of four first-line drugs given over a period of six to nine months. MDR-TB, however, usually must be treated longer, about eighteen months to two years. Even then, because second-line drugs must be used, the cure rate is not as good as with ordinary TB. It is about 50 to 70 percent. Although it is rare, people in the First World still die from MDR-TB. By preventing MDR-TB from being developed and spread, doctors are also preventing unnecessary deaths.

DOT: Curing Index Cases

About 1 percent of TB victims refuse to take their disease seriously and do not take their medications regularly. This is sometimes a problem with homeless people, alcoholics, drug

After Hurricane Katrina

When hurricane Katrina struck the Gulf Coast on August 29, 2005, 130 people in the New Orleans area were undergoing treatment for tuberculosis. Then people were evacuated, and hospitals and treatment centers were destroyed. The Louisiana TB Control headquarters had to be abandoned. Working from other areas, the TB staff had to track every known TB patient and ensure that each treatment was completed successfully. By September 21 the health workers had found 44 people living in their original homes. Their treatments could be resumed. Fourteen more people had been in prison and were not only safe but had continued their treatment regimens uninterrupted. Thirty-four patients were found through contacts with other state health departments that were providing TB treatment for displaced victims. These people had gone on their own to public health departments and asked for TB medicines. The last 38 people were difficult to find. The American Red Cross helped find 6. Other relief agencies identified 26 more. Six people were found when the Louisiana staff contacted pharmacies in the states where they were living and matched their names to the names on the Louisiana list. These people were voluntarily taking their medicines and cooperating with treatment programs, but Louisiana workers had to be sure. By October 13, 2005, every TB patient from New Orleans had been located and every patient was receiving appropriate treatment once again.

abusers, and the mentally ill. Public health workers use a system of "directly observed therapy," or DOT, to ensure that the noncompliant people are properly treated. This means that a public health or outreach worker watches a TB patient take his or her medicine every day until the patient is cured. It is not an easy job. Darryl Kilgore, an outreach worker at the New Jersey Medical School National Tuberculosis Center explains, "The first step is to establish rapport and trust with the client."[43]

One of Kilgore's clients, whom he called "Ken," was a homeless man who abused drugs, had HIV, and also suffered from pulmonary tuberculosis. Kilgore made friends with Ken and convinced him that taking his TB medicines was very important. Ken had had family members who died of TB, and he told Kilgore he did not want to die. Then Kilgore made friends with all Ken's friends and relatives so that they could help him find Ken when he moved from place to place. Kilgore searched Ken out and followed him around with the daily medicines in hand. "For one month," remembers Kilgore,

> I visited a dilapidated housing project where Ken stayed in an abandoned apartment along with other homeless substance abusers. He [Ken] described his housing as a "shooting gallery," a place in which he and others injected intravenous drugs. Every Monday through Friday, I would visit this drug-infested complex at 10 am and wait for Ken

Using directly observed therapy (DOT), a public health worker in South Africa watches a TB patient take his medication.

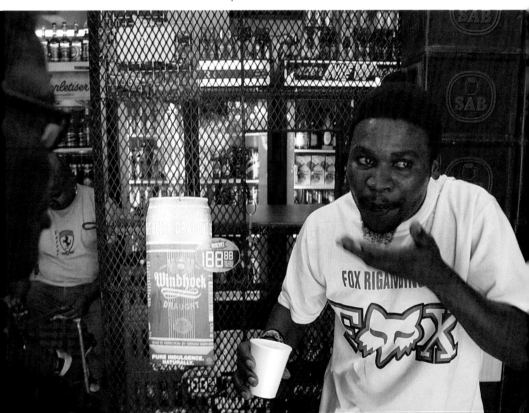

to emerge to take his medicine. Sometimes Ken would be there, and other times I might have to wait. I would watch the drug transactions taking place to pass time.[44]

Ken got sick and had to go to the hospital during the last two months of his treatment, but Kilgore visited him there, too. By the time Ken's DOT treatment was finished, not only was his tuberculosis cured, but he had also come to see Kilgore as his friend. Friendship and trust is the goal of all public health workers who provide DOT treatment. After about two weeks of TB treatment, patients are no longer infectious and can be free in the community as long as they continue to take their medicines. Outreach workers such as Kilgore make it possible for people with active TB to live in the community while friends and neighbors are protected from a TB outbreak. DOT treatment is very effective in societies that can afford the cost of hiring outreach workers and providing free of charge the expensive tuberculosis medicines needed to cure the disease.

As a Last Resort

Sometimes, however, TB patients are not as cooperative as Ken was, and directly observed therapy is not enough. Occasionally, legal intervention is necessary to protect society from a person with active TB. Most First World countries, including the United States, have court procedures that can order the detention of TB patients in hospitals until their treatments are complete.

Reichman and McDonald had one such patient whom they identify as "Maria." Maria had MDR-TB because, over the years, she had begun treatment several times and then forgotten her pills and gone on with her life. She was a high school drop-out who abused drugs and alcohol and had become a petty criminal. She just did not believe that TB was serious or important. Other hospitals had given up on Maria, but McDonald admitted her to a special isolation room, determined to cure her and prevent her MDR-TB from escaping into the community. Maria was cooperative at first, but her cooperation did not last. Says Reichman,

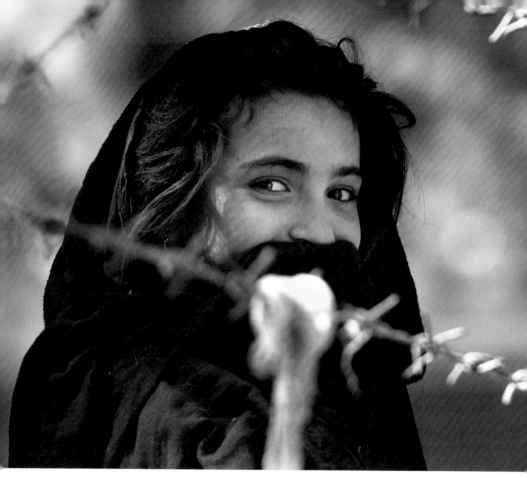

Despite having TB, a patient smiles as she stands in a fenced isolation area outside a hospital in Pakistan.

The drugs McDonald administered were second-line drugs (since Maria was resistant to the first-line drugs), and they had nasty side effects. After 2 months in an isolation room (which was costing the hospital $600 a day), Maria was not happy. Who could blame her? Even with television and a telephone, her life was acutely boring. She wanted to sign herself out against medical advice.[45]

McDonald had to get a restraining order to keep Maria in the hospital. Maria was not allowed to leave the hospital, and a guard was posted outside her hospital room to prevent her from doing so. She was so ill that eventually her doctors had to perform surgery and remove one of her destroyed lungs. After Maria recovered from the surgery, McDonald and Reichman decided to try sending her to her brother's home to finish her TB treatment. They were quite worried but hoped that it would work.

Finally, Maria took her TB seriously, but not because of the operation. Her brother showed her a newspaper story about another MDR-TB patient in New York who was extremely sick. It was as if a bell went off in her head. Maria said, "You mean this could happen to me if I don't take my medications? I might die?"[46] At last Maria became a cooperative patient and completed her treatment with no more problems. She was cured, and her family and friends were protected from the spread of MDR-TB.

MDR-TB and AIDS

Most people with MDR-TB are well aware of how grave the illness can be and how dangerous it is to others. They take their medicines willingly, no matter how difficult. Especially for people with AIDS, living with TB is a frightening struggle. John White, for example, is an Irish citizen who contracted AIDS when he was doing church work in Africa. He has survived AIDS for thirteen years. He became an AIDS advocate and worked for a European AIDS organization in London where he counseled other AIDS victims. One of White's clients was diagnosed with MDR-TB, and White discovered within six months of his contact with the client that he was a secondary case. White later said, "Here the nightmare begins! Here the greatest challenge in my 53 years of life began."[47]

After his MDR-TB was diagnosed, White spent six weeks in an isolation room in a London hospital. On the advice of public health doctors, he spent the next six weeks isolated in his home. Not even a visiting nurse could come into his house nor could any friends or family. Because his TB was resistant to first-line drugs, his treatment was very difficult. White explains,

> I endured taking four major TB drugs, plus intra-muscular injections of streptomycin, initially every day, later three times per week for one year. The entire time on medication I suffered extreme fatigue, constant skin problems, lethargy, sleeplessness, and lived with the constant fear

that at any time I may again test positive, i.e., the current drugs may prove [ineffective]. This would mean the nightmare beginning all over again.[48]

Fortunately, the drugs that White was given were able to overcome his resistant bacteria, and his weakened immune system did not prevent a cure of his tuberculosis.

White's experience is typical of the terrible ordeal that people with AIDS must endure when they are exposed to MDR-TB. Yet, despite his suffering, White was lucky that he lived in a country where TB outbreaks are diligently fought and appropriate medication is available. People in poor, developing countries often face a losing battle against tuberculosis, especially if they are also infected with HIV/AIDS. In many countries, living with TB is really dying of TB.

CHAPTER FIVE

TB Warriors for the Third World

Médecins Sans Frontières (MSF) is an international organization dedicated to fighting death and disease in Third World countries. In English, the organization is called Doctors Without Borders. The MSF Web site featured a headline in 2005; it said: "March 24 Is World Tuberculosis Day. To Mark the Occasion 5,000 People Are Going to Die."[49] Organizations such as Doctors Without Borders and the United Nations' World Health Organization (WHO) are trying to prevent the unending cycle of epidemic and death in developing countries where someone dies of TB every ten seconds. Public health systems to control TB's spread do not exist in these places. Money for expensive, long-term treatments and drugs is unavailable. Hospitals where patients can recover and be prevented from infecting others are few. Education and understanding of tuberculosis transmission is very low. Still, dedicated doctors and TB health workers are determined to bring the breakthroughs of the First World to the people of the Third World. They hope to raise the awareness and consciousness of the rich countries so that the battle against TB can be won.

DOT, with an S

In 1993 WHO declared tuberculosis to be a global emergency and recommended directly observed therapy, short course

(DOTS) as the way to reduce epidemics in developing countries. The theory is that a standard six- to eight-month treatment program that includes directly observing patients swallow their medicine will lead to cure rates of almost 80 percent. Thus, the infectious spread of TB to others can be slowed, and the number of people with tuberculosis within each country can be reduced by about 6 percent per year. At the same time, because people are observed taking their medicine, MDR-TB strains cannot develop. Eventually, WHO planners believe that this approach will lead to the disappearance of TB epidemics.

DOTS is a strategy for protecting public health and doing the greatest good for the greatest number of people. Therefore, the strategy concentrates on what is practical in poverty-stricken countries, rather than treating all who are sick or in danger. It is a treatment method only for those with infectious, easily diagnosed TB—that is, active pulmonary tuberculosis.

A Turkish TB patient waits to be treated in a clinic run by Médecins Sans Frontiéres (Doctors Without Borders).

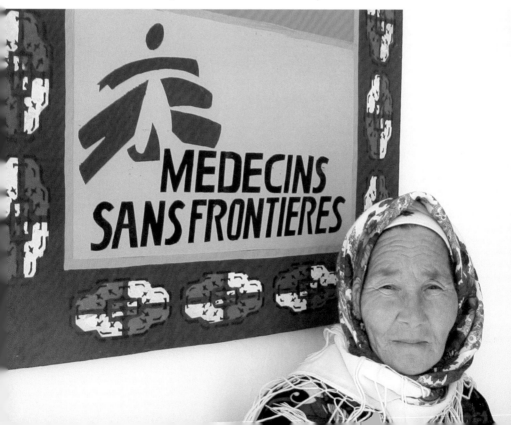

To Make DOTS Work

The World Health Organization's DOTS strategy is based on five basic principles:

1. The government of the country of operation must agree to be committed to long-term TB control programs.

2. Every person who comes to a treatment facility with symptoms must have a sputum test.

3. In people who test smear-positive for pulmonary TB, treatment must last six to eight months with Directly Observed Therapy (DOT) for the first two months (the short part).

4. Health workers and doctors must be provided with a regular, uninterrupted supply of all essential TB medicines.

5. All results must be recorded and reported so that WHO can assess the success and value of its TB control program in each country.

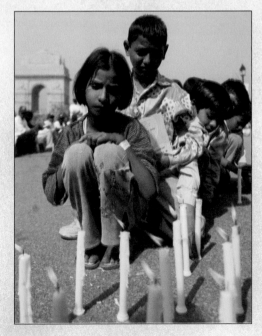

Young TB patients in New Delhi, India, light candles to mark World Tuberculosis Day.

TB is easily diagnosed when a test of a victim's sputum is smear-positive. In other words, if TB bacteria in a smear of sputum are seen under a microscope, the patient is diagnosed with TB and treated. Otherwise, however, in the DOTS approach, a sick person is not treated. Often TB cases cannot be diagnosed with this simple test, but more sophisticated tests are not possible in the developing world. The result is that many sick people are left out.

Not for Everyone

People with TB in organs other than lungs (in bones, blood, etc.) do not have smear-positive sputum and so are not treated. Since this extrapulmonary TB is not usually infectious, treating it, according to the DOTS theory, has no effect on stopping the spread of TB. Often pulmonary TB victims are not smear-positive either. People who are very sick and weak, for example, may not cough strongly enough to bring up bacteria. Children usually are unable to cough up sputum. These victims, also, are not treated since they are not infectious to others. People with MDR-TB are not treated because a short course is not worthwhile, and it is assumed that these people will die anyway.

Despite the TB sufferers who are omitted from DOTS programs, DOTS has been very successful in many countries at reducing the incidence of TB in populations as a whole. It is in operation in 192 countries and has decreased epidemics and new infections in many of them. Most doctors and scientists, however, are badly disturbed by the strategy. MSF, for example, argues, "The overall result is that smear-negative, extrapulmonary, and pediatric TB patients continue to be second-class citizens in the management of TB."[50] In response to such criticism, WHO expanded its DOTS strategy in 2002 and specifically stated that every person has the right to TB care. In practice, however, achieving this right is not easy. Even MSF refused to try to treat TB infections when it was organized thirty years ago because of its fear of causing MDR-TB in places where people could not be monitored daily and treated for months. Today, MSF uses DOTS strategies along with some very creative programs to try to bring modern treatments to places in the Third World.

Mado

In 2001, in the Afar region of Ethiopia, MSF built a "patient village" in a town called Galaha. In this village, four hundred huts called *daboytas* are available for patients at MSF's Galaha TB center. People who are sick with TB can stay in the village until their treatment is complete. While they are there, both food and medicine are provided free of charge. Those who are very sick receive extra portions of milk. In an area the size of California, the Galaha TB Center is the only clinic offering TB care. The Afar people are nomads, who travel the region with their animals searching for food and water. Yet, many find their way to the Galaha TB center. One such sufferer was a fifty-two-year-old man named Mado. He said, "I got the 'coughing disease.'. . . I live in the desert with my herd of goats and travel from one water site to the next. There are no health clinics near where I live, but I had heard that there was a hospital in a small village called Galaha that provided free treatment."[51] Mado sold a goat to pay for his trip, got a friend to care for his animals, and traveled for a day and a half to get to the MSF hospital. The trip was not easy; Mado had to hobble with a crutch because one of his feet had been bitten off by a crocodile when he was young.

When Mado arrived at the village he was diagnosed with pulmonary tuberculosis and admitted to the center. For four months he lived in a hut there while he took his daily TB medications under direct observation. Then, after receiving education about the importance of continuing the treatment, he was given three more months' worth of medicines to take at home. Mado's treatment was successful because the MSF DOTS approach met his needs. He was not expected to travel dozens of miles every day to take his medicine in front of a health worker. He lived only a few feet away from the hospital in his *daboyta*. A medical coordinator at Galaha says, "MSF is successful in treating the Afar nomads because [it] provides for patients to live near the clinic throughout the intensive phase

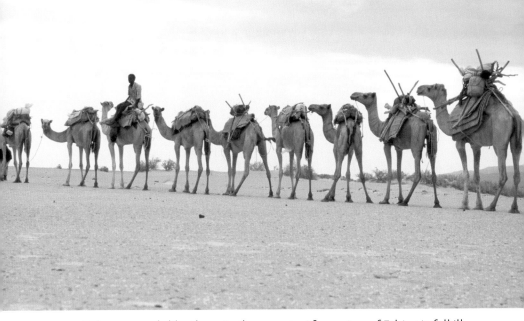

When nomads like these in the remote Afar region of Ethiopia fall ill, they often seek medical help at the Galaha TB Center.

of their treatment regimen. . . . Imagine telling people whose livelihood depends on being with their animals that they have to go to a health facility every day for six months to take your drugs."[52] Mado did not depend on his animals while he lived in the village. The Galaha TB center provided for him.

Mayram

The Galaha TB center does not turn TB patients away. Mayram, for example, was a twenty-two-year-old woman with extrapulmonary TB. That meant that the smear of her sputum was negative. Yet, Mayram was so weak that her brother had to bring her to the hospital since she could not walk alone. It was hard for doctors to diagnose her, because the lab tests for diagnosing extrapulmonary TB are too sophisticated and expensive for a small Ethiopian clinic. Still, the doctors wanted to do their best to help her. Mayram says,

> I had been coughing for five months, had night fever, experiencing a lot of chest pain, and feeling very, very weak. I couldn't even go to the toilet by myself. My husband left

me when he found out I was sick with TB. He also took our two-year-old daughter with him. My other child died when she was three and a half months old. I thought I would die from being sick and die from sadness.[53]

Mayram moved into the TB village, and doctors began treatment for her tuberculosis despite not knowing which medicines would be best to treat her. After only ten days her cough and chest pain disappeared. She needed to stay at the village for eight months for her difficult treatment, but she did not mind. She explains, "MSF is very good to give us food, a place to live, doctors, and medicines for free, so I can stay."[54]

Ricardo

MSF's village strategy for TB treatment is used not just in Ethiopia but in other poor countries, too. In Angola, for example, the district hospital in the town of Kuito joined with MSF to build living quarters for TB patients and their families. The roads in this war-torn country are much too dangerous for daily travel to a hospital, even though a peace agreement is in place. People who are admitted to the TB treatment program understand that they must promise to stay for many months until their disease is cured. Ricardo, for instance, was a boy soldier in Angola who developed active tuberculosis when he was twenty-one. He had never heard of tuberculosis. He just knew that he found it hard to breathe and walk and was coughing up blood. Some villagers told him about TB and the Kuito hospital. Ricardo had to stay at the hospital for eight months, but he did not mind. Like many desperately poor people, he was better off there than anywhere else. He said, "I get a meal here three times a day, I have a bed to sleep in and I've made some friends, I'm much more afraid of the future: once the treatment is finished."[55]

Nonkululo

In South Africa MSF faces a worse problem than poverty-stricken, homeless patients with no place to go. South Africa has a dual epidemic of HIV/AIDS and tuberculosis. Together with the South African government, MSF has started the Ubuntu clinic in Khayelitsha, a township near Cape Town, where people with both diseases can be treated. More than two hundred people come to the Ubuntu clinic every day, either to be tested or treated for their infections. Sixty-five percent of all the TB patients at Ubuntu are HIV positive. Nonkululo Kili became one of those patients when she was diagnosed as HIV positive in 2000. She remembers, "I was very, very sick. I had headache. I went to the clinic and the doctor tested me for HIV and it was yes. I had to cry and cry." When the clinic tested Kili for tuberculosis, the doctors discovered that she had TB also. Kili took TB medicines for eight months and was given antiretroviral medicines for HIV, which got the HIV under control. Then by 2003, Kili was cured of tuberculosis. She acquired a job at Ubuntu clinic as a cleaner. She says, "Inside I'm feeling so good. The TB is gone. Now while I'm working I see people who are very sick, who have the same problems. I talk to these people. I tell them that I was sick too. And now I'm working every day."[56]

A woman and her baby await treatment at a tuberculosis clinic in Kuito, Angola.

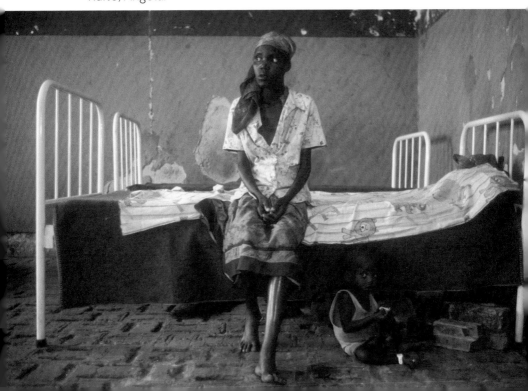

Kili was treated at Ubuntu with a flexible DOTS strategy. She and all Ubuntu clients are given counseling so they can understand the importance of completing TB treatment. A treatment buddy was assigned to her to help her keep up with the medication schedule. She was directly observed as she took her medicines for several weeks and then was trusted to take her medicines at home and come to the clinic for checkups.

Drops in the Ocean

Kili's experience was a success story. Combining treatment for both TB and HIV worked for her and for many others at Ubuntu. However, as MSF worker Lisa Hayes says, "Ubuntu is one of only a handful of South African health centers that are offering integrated care for TB and HIV patients and all these efforts pale in comparison to the immense need for them."[57]

Near death from AIDS when she first visited the MSF Ubuntu clinic in Khayelitsha, South Africa, this young woman is now healthy.

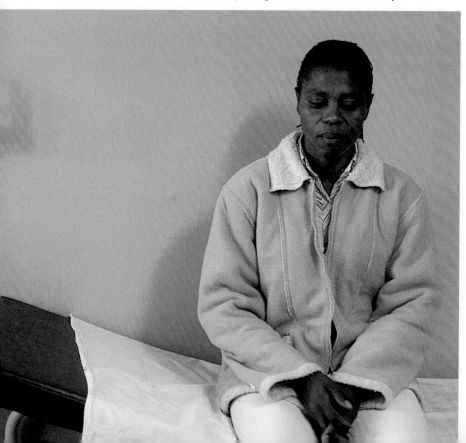

Many people with TB are not treated at all, either because they have no access to care or because their sputum is smear-negative. HIV-positive people often test negative for TB bacteria. Their bodies are so weak that they cannot cough up enough sputum and bacteria to find under a microscope. Or they have extrapulmonary TB, which is increasing due to HIV/AIDS. At Ubuntu, these people, and children with TB, are always given TB medication if doctors feel they have symptoms of TB. Some die anyway, but many patients in this little corner of South Africa are saved.

MSF doctors are frustrated that they cannot reach more people and do more to prevent the deadly spread of TB in people who are HIV positive, and they worry about the future. Says physician Shaheed Matee, "We treat our patients for six months, and then we have to send them back to the same conditions where they got it the first time. They go back to the overcrowding, the lack of sanitation, no water, no electricity, that type of thing. So there are social issues that have to be looked at before we can even say we are going to get TB under control."[58] Matee says many of the cured patients can be reinfected with TB when they go home again. The social conditions that cause TB to erupt in poor countries are of grave concern to MSF workers all over the world.

The Worst of the Worst

In Abkhazia, a republic in Georgia (once part of the Soviet Union), MSF runs a program to treat people with MDR-TB. The republic is very poor and has little social or medical care available for its citizens. Between 2001 and 2005 MSF treated eighty-nine people with MDR-TB in its hospital. Thirteen of these patients were cured; forty-five are still being treated; but the rest have either died or left the program before treatment was completed. A large problem for MSF workers in Abkhazia is that the treatment for MDR-TB is so long and so terrible that people refuse to continue it. Physician Cathy Hewison explains, "The length of the treatment makes it extremely difficult. But most of all, it's important to realize that it's as drastic and toxic as chemotherapy used against cancer."[59]

To treat MDR-TB, the patient must swallow four second-line drugs each day and be given painful daily injections for at least six months. For the next eighteen months, the tablets alone are taken twice a day. Most patients have to live in or near the hospital for all this time. They cannot go back home or see their families. Moreover, many of the second-line drugs cause painful, distressing side effects. People develop serious nausea and inability to eat. Joint pains and kidney or liver damage can occur. One of the drugs can even cause depression and mental illness. Hewison remembers, "One of our patients sliced open his stomach with a knife because he thought a monster was inside it."[60] It is little wonder that the cure rate for MDR-TB is low, even with the best treatments provided by MSF. Worldwide, less than half of all people with MDR-TB ever recover.

Nevertheless, MSF continues its efforts. In about twenty-four different developing countries MSF runs TB projects that aim to help every TB patient who seeks treatment. In most of these situations they have discovered that flexibility in treatment programs and new ways to diagnose and treat TB are needed. WHO has agreed with this assessment. Millions still die of extrapulmonary TB, MDR-TB, and TB plus HIV/AIDS, and MSF and WHO reach just a small percentage of infected people in limited areas of each country.

A New Plan to Stop TB

The Stop TB Partnership is a global movement, led by WHO, that includes more than four hundred partners, such as governments, private institutions, companies, individuals, and donors who are dedicated to fighting TB around the world. The partnership supports more than the DOTS strategy to stop TB. It advocates an expanded, flexible DOTS approach, as recommended by MSF, to improve public health around the world, and it promotes the development of new, more powerful, and more affordable treatments and tests for tuberculosis. On January 27, 2006, the Stop TB Partnership announced the Global Plan to Stop TB, 2006–2015. The goal is to raise $51 billion by 2015 for TB treatment and research and to move toward a world free of tuberculosis by 2050.

A TB Vaccine

A vaccine to help prevent TB was developed decades ago and is still used in Europe. It is called BCG vaccine and is given to many infants and children in European countries. The vaccine seems better than nothing to European doctors because it works well to protect children from tubercular meningitis. Experts say the vaccine's protection wears off and its effectiveness is limited. In the United States, doctors and health officials never used the BCG vaccine because they consider it of little value. Still, most doctors believe that TB will never be eradicated or even controlled without an effective vaccine. Developing a new TB vaccine is a major goal of the Stop TB Partnership.

In March 2006 in Rockville, Maryland, the Aeras Global TB Vaccine Foundation opened its first factory to produce TB vaccine—even though no such vaccine has been invented. The chief executive officer and vaccine developer Jerald Sadoff explains that researchers, supported by the Bill and Melinda Gates Foundation, are working on a new vaccine, and the factory is waiting for success. In an interview Sadoff says, "In private industry you really have to start building your factory early. . . . You need to be able to do your clinical trials with the final product. So we can have all that ready. . . . With more than 4,700 people dying every day from TB, the world needs an effective TB vaccine as soon as possible. This new facility can deliver a TB vaccine to the world as soon as one is available." Sadoff says his factory will be able to produce 150 million doses a year when the vaccine is developed, but that will probably take another seven to ten years of work.

Jerald Sadoff, interview by Reuters, *MSNBC*. www.msnbc.msn.com/id/11982114.

Marcos Espinal, the executive secretary of the Stop TB Partnership, describes the goals of the global plan:

> We will treat 50 million people with TB, cure 90% of them and save the lives of an additional 14 million people—the vast majority of them working adults in low income countries.

We will put 3 million TB patients co-infected with HIV onto antiretrovirals by testing and counseling for HIV in national TB programmes.

We will end the death sentence imposed by multidrug-resistant TB by massively scaling up treatment to nearly a million patients over 10 years.

We will deliver the first new TB drug in 40 years by 2010, which will shorten treatment and help reduce the spread of drug resistance.

We will deliver a new point-of-service diagnostic [an easy field test for diagnosing TB] by 2010, which will be fast, affordable, and effective in detecting TB infection in HIV [positive] people.

We will deliver by 2015 the first new TB vaccine since the early 1900s. . . .

In summary, with this Plan, these powerful new tools, and the resources to do the job, we will break the back of the global TB epidemic and create the conditions to eliminate tuberculosis as a public health problem by 2050.[61]

Persuading the World to Care

The global plan is ambitious and far-reaching, and will require the help of many First World countries. It will need about $5.5 billion each year to spend on treatment and research in order to meet the goals. At the international meeting where Espinal announced the plan, Great Britain pledged $74.63 million to fight TB in India. Bill Gates announced that the Gates Foundation would contribute $900 million for research and the development of new drugs and TB tests. He and other members of the Stop TB Partnership called on world leaders to join in the fight against TB. By the spring of 2006, however, less than half the money that Stop TB needs had been promised by developed countries.

Archbishop Desmond Tutu asked all the people of the world to support the Global Plan to Stop TB. He said,

I know how debilitating this disease can be. I contracted TB at the age of 14 and was hospitalized for 20 months.

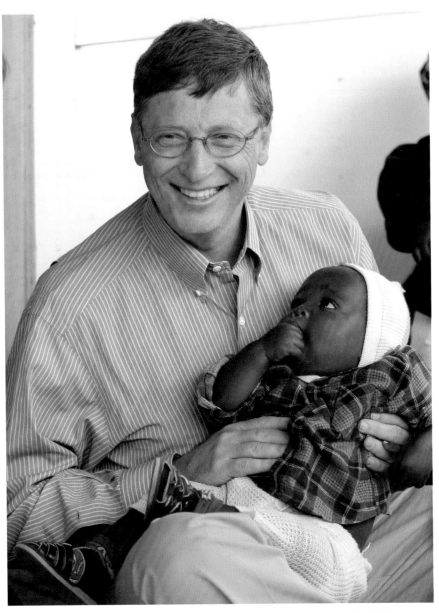

The Gates Foundation, created by Bill Gates (pictured in Africa), has pledged $900 million to the global effort to eradicate TB.

I'm here to witness that TB is a curable and preventable disease. . . . Treating patients and saving lives is a moral and ethical imperative. We need you to help; we have a global partnership, a global strategy, and a new Global Plan; help us to stop TB![62]

Notes

Introduction: A Renewed Battle Against an Old Enemy

1. Lee B. Reichman with Janice Hopkins Tanne, *Timebomb: The Global Epidemic of Multi-Drug-Resistant Tuberculosis*. New York: McGraw-Hill, 2002, p. 216.
2. Frank Ryan, *The Forgotten Plague: How the Battle Against Tuberculosis Was Won—And Lost*. Boston: Little, Brown, 1993, p. 416.

Chapter 1: What Is Tuberculosis?

3. Ryan, The *Forgotten Plague*, p. 22.
4. Ryan, *The Forgotten Plague*, p. 22.
5. Quoted in Reichman, *Timebomb*, p. 18.
6. Reichman, *Timebomb*, p. 168.
7. Ryan, *The Forgotten Plague*, p. 23.
8. Stanley B. Burns, "A Photo History of Women's Health: Nonpulmonary Complications of Tuberculosis," *Women's Health in Primary Care*, vol. 8, no. 8, September 2005. www.womenshealthpc.com/09_05/pdfs/402Photohistory.pdf.
9. Ryan, *The Forgotten Plague*, p. 23.
10. Ryan, *The Forgotten Plague*, p. 19.
11. Reichman, *Timebomb*, pp. 13–14.
12 Quoted in Reichman, *Timebomb*, p. 151.
13. Quoted in Reichman, *Timebomb*, p. 152.
14. Quoted in Reichman, *Timebomb*, p. 11.

Chapter 2: Deadly Mystery

15. Quoted in Nobelprize.org, "Robert Koch and Tuberculosis." http://nobelprize.org/medicine/educational/tuberculosis/readmore.html.
16. Quoted in Ryan, *The Forgotten Plague*, pp. 14–15.

17. Quoted in Nobelprize.org, "Robert Koch and Tuberculosis."
18. Quoted in Thomas Dormandy, *The White Death: A History of Tuberculosis*. New York: New York University Press, 2000, p. 367.
19. Quoted in Dormandy, *The White Death*, p. 178.
20 Quoted in Dormandy, *The White Death*, p. 179.
21. Quoted in John F. Murray, "Bill Dock and the Location of Pulmonary Tuberculosis: How Bed Rest Might Have Helped Consumption," *American Journal of Respiratory and Critical Care Medicine*, November 1, 2003. www.find articles.com/p/articles/mi_qa4085/is_200311/ai_n93256120.
22. Quoted in Sing365.Com, Merle Haggard Lyrics: "T.B. Blues" Lyrics. www.sing365.com/music/lyric.nsf/T-B-Blues-lyrics-Merle-Haggard/C2A123AD704E618348256 D91002CC131.
23. Quoted in Ryan, *The Forgotten Plague*, pp. 220–21.
24. Quoted in Ryan, *The Forgotten Plague*, p. 239.
25. Quoted in Ryan, *The Forgotten Plague*, p. 276.
26. Quoted in Ryan, *The Forgotten Plague*, p. 277.

Chapter 3: The Disease That Fought Back

27. Quoted in Reichman, *Timebomb*, p. 10.
28. John F. Murray, "A Century of Tuberculosis," *American Journal of Respiratory and Critical Care Medicine*, vol. 169, 2004, http://ajrccm.atsjournals.org/cgi/content/full/169/11/1181.
29. Quoted in Reichman, *Timebomb*, p. 43.
30. Reichman, *Timebomb*, pp. 44–45.
31. Quoted in Reichman, *Timebomb*, p. 47.
32. Quoted in Ryan, *The Forgotten Plague*, p. 393.
33. Murray, "A Century of Tuberculosis."
34. Quoted in Moscow Helsinki Group, "Tuberculosis in Russian Prisons: Dying for Reform." www.mhg.ru/english /1F11E20.
35. Quoted in Moscow Helsinki Group, "Tuberculosis in Russian Prisons."
36. Quoted in *Medical News Today*, "Russia—Untreatable Tuberculosis Boom?" January 27, 2004. www.medical

newstoday.com/medicalnews.php?newsid=5544.

37. Quoted in Ryan, *The Forgotten Plague*, p. 403.
38. Dormandy, *The White Death*, p. 386.

Chapter 4: Combating TB in the First World

39. Rupert, "Welcome to Rupert's Story," UK Coalition of People Living with HIV & AIDS. www.ukcoalition.org/tb/rupertstory.htm.
40. Alexandria, "Welcome to Alexandria's Story," UK Coalition of People Living with HIV & AIDS. www.uk coalition.org/tb/alexstory.htm.
41. Reichman, *Timebomb*, pp. 135, 136.
42. Reichman, *Timebomb*, p. 131.
43. Quoted in Khalil Sabu Rashidi and Debra Bottinick, "Making Directly Observed Therapy Work," NJMS National Tuberculosis Center, 2001. www.umdnj.edu/ntbcweb/tb_frame.html.
44. Quoted in Rashidi and Bottinick, "Making Directly Observed Therapy Work."
45. Reichman, *Timebomb*, p. 164.
46. Quoted in Reichman, *Timebomb*, p. 170.
47. John White, "Welcome to John White's Story," UK Coalition of People Living with HIV & AIDS. www.ukcoalition. org /tb/jwstory.htm.
48. White, "Welcome to John White's Story."

Chapter 5: TB Warriors for the Third World

49. Médecins Sans Frontières, "TB Care in Kuito, Angola: Three Interviews," March 24, 2005. www.msf.org/msfin ternational/invoke.cfm?component=article&objectid= 477C42AB-E018-0C72-0971F0CA1BC7E0EE&method =full_html.
50. Laura Hakokongas, ed., "Running Out of Breath: TB Care in the 21st Century," *MSF Activity Report*, Médecins Sans Frontières, March, 2005. www.doctorswithoutborders. org/publications/reports/2005/tbreport_2005.pdf.
51. Quoted in Médecins Sans Frontières, "Treating Ethiopian Nomads Living with Tuberculosis," August 22, 2005.

www.doctorswithoutborders.org/news/2005/08-22-2005_1.htm.

52. Quoted in Médecins Sans Frontières, "Treating Ethiopian Nomads."

53. Quoted in Médecins Sans Frontières, "Treating Ethiopian Nomads."

54. Quoted in Médecins Sans Frontières, "Treating Ethiopian Nomads."

55. Quoted in Médecins Sans Frontières, "TB Care in Kuito, Angola."

56. Quoted in Lisa Hayes, "The TB/HIV Time Bomb: A Dual Epidemic Explodes in South Africa," *International Activity Report*, Médecins Sans Frontières, 2005. www.doctorswithoutborders.org/publications/ar/i2005/article_tbhiv.cfm.

57. Hayes, "The TB/HIV Time Bomb."

58. Quoted in Hayes, "The TB/HIV Time Bomb."

59. Quoted in Médecins Sans Frontières, "Multidrug-Resistant Tuberculosis: No Tools to Properly Treat People," October 11, 2005. www.doctorswithout borders.org/news/2005/10-11-2005_1.htm.

60. Quoted in Médecins Sans Frontières, "Multidrug-Resistant Tuberculosis."

61. Marcos Espinal, "Speech of Dr. Marcos Espinal, Executive Secretary, Stop TB Partnership at the Global Plan to Stop TB," press conference, Davos, Switzerland, January 27, 2006; repr., Global Plan to Stop TB, 2006–2015, Stop TB Partnership. www.stoptb.org/globalplan/assets/docu ments/Davos%20speech%20Marcos.pdf.

62. Desmond Tutu, "Archbishop Desmond Tutu on the Global Plan to Stop TB," video transcript, Global Plan Supporters, Global Plan to Stop TB, 2006–2015, Stop TB Partnership. www.stoptb.org/globalplan/assets/documents/Archbishop%20Desmond%20Tutu%20on%20the%20Global%20Plan%20to%20Stop%20TB.pdf.

Glossary

active tuberculosis: A tuberculosis infection that has developed into actual disease. The body has not successfully fought the bacteria which are able to grow and multiply. Active tuberculosis is infectious to others.

AIDS: Acquired immunodeficiency syndrome; an infectious disease caused by the human immunodeficiency virus (HIV).

antibiotic: A drug used to treat bacterial infections.

bacillus: Any bacterium with a rodlike shape. Tuberculosis bacteria are members of the large family of rod-shaped bacteria.

bacterium: A single-celled microscopic organism that can live independently, as in soil, or may live as a parasite dependent on another life form, such as an animal or a human.

consumption: The historical term for pulmonary tuberculosis.

DNA: Deoxyribonucleic acid; the hereditary material that encodes genetic information and determines the development of every living thing.

DOTS: Directly observed therapy, short course. It is the internationally recommended treatment strategy for controlling TB and includes directly observing the patient taking prescribed drugs over a specific period of time.

epidemic: A sudden outbreak of a disease that involves more cases of the disease than expected in a given area in a specific time.

extrapulmonary tuberculosis: Tuberculosis that occurs outside the lungs.

hemorrhage: Bleeding, especially excessive bleeding.

immune system: The complex system in the body that protects it from infections and foreign substances by seeking out and destroying invaders.

latent tuberculosis: Tuberculosis infection that is dormant, causes no symptoms, and is not infectious to others.

macrophage: A specialized white blood cell of the immune system that eats foreign invaders.

MDR-TB: Multidrug-resistant tuberculosis; any strain of tuberculosis that does not respond to two or more standard anti-TB drugs.

Mycobacterium tuberculosis: The scientific name of the bacterium that causes tuberculosis; sometimes called *M. tuberculosis.*

parasite: An organism that lives in or on another organism and is dependent upon that organism for its survival.

petri dish: A shallow, circular dish used in laboratories to grow bacteria and other microorganisms.

phthisis: An old name for tuberculosis. Pronounced TEE-sis or TIE-sis.

pulmonary: Of the lungs.

sanatorium: A long-term recuperation and rest facility for people who are chronically ill. Sanatoria became standard treatment for tuberculosis victims in the late nineteenth and early twentieth centuries.

smear-positive: Bacterial growth identified on a microscopic slide of a sputum sample.

sputum: Matter coughed up from the lungs, including mucus, pus, blood, bacterial substances, and other foreign matter.

tubercle: A small, hard lump that is like a tumor or boil and is the characteristic symptom of active tuberculosis.

Organizations to Contact

American Lung Association
61 Broadway, 6th Floor, New York, NY 10006
(800) LUNGUSA
www.lungusa.org/site/pp.asp?c=dvLUK9O0E&b=22542

The American Lung Association is dedicated to preventing all lung diseases, including tuberculosis. There is a link at the Web site to contact your local chapter.

CDC: National Center for HIV, STD, and TB Prevention
(800) 232-4636
e-mail: CDCINFO@cdc.gov
www.cdc.gov/nchstp/tb/contact.htm

The U.S. Centers for Disease Control provide general information about TB prevention, treatment, and research.

Stop TB Partnership
Stop TB Partnership Secretariat, World Health Organization, HTM/STB/TBP, 20, Avenue Appia, CH-1211 Geneva, 27 Switzerland
+(41) 22 791 2708
e-mail: info@stoptb.org
www.stoptb.org/contact.asp

This global organization, led by WHO, provides a wealth of information about tuberculosis and strategies to fight and control the disease.

UKC: UK Coalition of People Living with HIV and AIDS
250 Kennington Lane, London SE11 5RD, England, UK
+44 (0) 20 7564 2180
fax: +44 (0) 20 7564 2140
e-mail: reception@ukcoalition.org
www.ukcoalition.org

This site includes a large section for people with AIDS who also have TB.

For Further Reading

Books

Deborah Ellis, *Our Stories, Our Songs: African Children Talk About AIDS*. Markham, ON: Fitzhenry and Whiteside, 2005. This is a sad book about the tragedy of AIDS in sub-Saharan Africa. Real African children tell their own stories about how their lives have been touched by the AIDS epidemic. Facts about AIDS and quotes from experts are included, too.

Betty MacDonald, *The Plague and I*. Pleasantville, NY: Akadine, 2000. This reissue of an old book is a witty and honest description of the author's sojourn in a TB sanatorium in 1938–1939.

Randy Shilts, *And the Band Played On: Politics, People and the AIDS Epidemic*. New York: St. Martin's, 1988. This best-selling book is the classic description of the AIDS epidemic and how it spread, not only from a medical point of view but especially how politics and culture fueled the crisis.

Gail B. Stewart, *Great Medical Discoveries: Tuberculosis*. San Diego: Lucent, 2002. Read about the history of tuberculosis treatments and the discovery of the first antibiotics, as well as the strategies that are needed to conquer TB in modern times.

Web Sites:

Dr. Selman Waksman (1888–1973) (www.scc.rutgers.edu/ njh/SciANDTech/Waksman/biog2.htm). This short biography from Rutgers University's Waksman Institute describes Selman Waksman's contributions to TB treatments and to medicine as a whole.

How the World Health Organization Works (http://people. howstuffworks.com/who.htm). Learn about WHO and the work it does to promote health throughout the developing world.

**Médecins Sans Frontières/Doctors Without Borders US
Section: Tuberculosis** (www.doctorswithoutborders.org/
news/tuberculosis/index.cfm). This site is continually up-
dated with news from around the world where MSF is working against TB and saving lives.

Robert Koch (www.historylearningsite.co.uk/robert_koch.
htm). Read a short biography of Robert Koch and learn
why he is considered so important to the advancement of
medicine.

TBTV (www.darbyfilms.com/client/tbtv). This is an activist,
global support group for people with tuberculosis. Read stories from people with TB and learn the latest TB news.

**World TB Day 2006: Actions for Life: Towards a World
Free of Tuberculosis** (www.stoptb.org/events/world_tb_
day/2006). Read the latest news about the world campaign
to stop TB; see the different events that took place in various countries on World TB day; download TB posters.

Index

Picture Credits

About the Author

Toney Allman holds degrees from Ohio State University and University of Hawaii. She currently lives in Virginia where she writes nonfiction books for students.